Essential Anatomy for Anesthesia

For Churchill Livingstone

Commissioning Editor: Gavin Smith
Project Manager: Nora Naughton
PTU: Gerard Heyburn
Copy Editor: Elizabeth Lightfoot
Indexer: Nina Boyd

Essential Anatomy for Anesthesia

Sue M. Black BSc PhD
Consultant Anatomist and Forensic Anthropologist,
Department of Forensic Medicine and Science,
University of Glasgow, Glasgow, UK

W. Alastair Chambers MD FRCA
Consultant in Anaesthesia and Pain Management,
Aberdeen Royal Hospitals, Foresterhill, Aberdeen;
Clinical Senior Lecturer, University of Aberdeen,
Aberdeen, UK

Illustrations by
Peter Cox

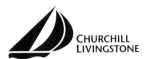

CHURCHILL LIVINGSTONE

New York Edinburgh London Madrid Melbourne San Francisco
and Tokyo 1997

CHURCHILL LIVINGSTONE
Medical Division of Pearson Professional Limited

Distributed in the United States of America by Churchill
Livingstone Inc., 650 Avenue of the Americas, New York,
N.Y. 10011, and by associated companies, branches and
representatives throughout the world.

First published 1997

ISBN 0 443 05054 6

British Library Cataloguing in Publication Data
A catalogue record for this book is available from the British
Library.

Library of Congress Cataloging in Publication Data
A catalog record for this book is available from the Library of
Congress.

Note
Medical knowledge is constantly changing. As new information
becomes available, changes in treatment, procedures, equipment
and the use of drugs become necessary. The authors and the
publishers have, as far as it is possible, taken care to ensure that
the information given in this text is accurate and up to date.
However, readers are strongly advised to confirm that the
information, especially with regard to drug usage, complies with
latest legislation and standards of practice.

Produced by Longman Asia Ltd, Hong Kong
CTPS/01

Contents

Preface

A sound knowledge of relevant anatomy remains a fundamental requirement for specialists in anesthesia. Although many of the essential areas have remained largely unchanged for many years, recent changes in practice such as increased involvement in the provision of local anesthesia for eye surgery have extended the requirements. This text aims to cover the areas required by those who wish to refresh their knowledge prior to learning procedures and by candidates for the fellowship examinations. It does not include detailed clinical application such as details of nerve blocks which are available in many excellent texts. Specialists and trainees should find the clinical application or the need to seek further information in specialist texts obvious. In any descriptive anatomy text, decisions have to be taken by the authors where to provide additional detail and where not and for the sake of consistency and completeness, certain sections do provide more information than might be necessary for examination candidates. Full use has been made of illustrations and tables to demonstrate and summarize important features. The interpretation of chest X-rays and the anatomical features of these are also included. However, more specialized imaging techniques normally require specialist interpretation and their inclusion would not have assisted in understanding the anatomy.

S.M.B.
W.A.C.

Acknowledgements

The authors wish to express their gratitude to Dr Louise Scheuer, Department of Anatomy and Developmental Biology, Royal Free Hospital School of Medicine, for her invaluable comments and criticisms throughout the production of this text.

S.M.B.
W.A.C

1

The respiratory system

Although this chapter is principally concerned with the respiratory system, it must by necessity also consider the upper regions of the alimentary tract as they share a common course, albeit for a relatively short distance. The respiratory system is separated into an upper and a lower respiratory tract with the former consisting of the nose and pharynx, and the latter consisting of the larynx, trachea and lungs.

THE NOSE

This is the most superior part of the upper respiratory tract and serves 3 important functions:

1. it filters, warms and humidifies air before transferring it to the lower regions of the respiratory tract
2. it houses the olfactory epithelium
3. it acts as a conducting channel for the removal and transfer of secretions from the paranasal air sinuses to the alimentary tract.

The **external nose** is an osteocartilaginous framework which forms a prominent feature of the face and can vary considerably both in size and shape (Fig. 1.1). It resembles a three-sided pyramid which opens to the exterior by paired nostrils or external nares that are separated by a midline nasal septum.

The bony skeleton forms the immovable areas of the nose and comprises paired nasal bones, the frontal processes of the maxillae and the nasal processes of the frontal bone, with the margins of these bones forming the piriform aperture. The movable cartilaginous area forms the greater part of the external nose and consists of 5 large pieces of hyaline cartilage and up to 8 minor cartilages. The boundaries of the external nares are formed from these cartilages and their shape can be altered by the action of the facial muscles.

The **vestibule** is the entrance to the nose and consists of a slight dilation immediately superior to the nostrils. It is lined with skin from which numerous hairs project and these help to filter the inspired air and remove foreign matter.

The **nasal cavity** is vertically divided by a nasal septum that is frequently deviated to one side, resulting in 2 cavities of unequal size. These open onto the face via the nostrils or external nares and communicate posteriorly with the nasopharynx via the internal nares or choanae.

In sagittal section the nasal cavities have a simple geometrical shape, with a floor, roof, vertical medial wall and sloping lateral walls (Figs. 1.2A and 1.2B). Each cavity is wider below than above and is both widest and highest in the central region. The **roof** is tent-shaped, as the anterior one-third slopes inferiorly and anteriorly, the middle third passes virtually

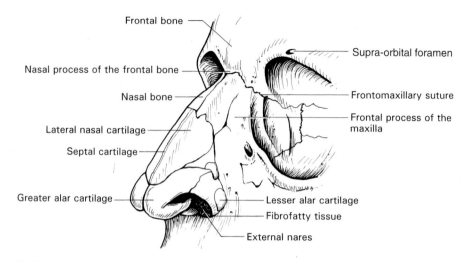

Fig. 1.1
Osteocartilaginous framework of the nose.

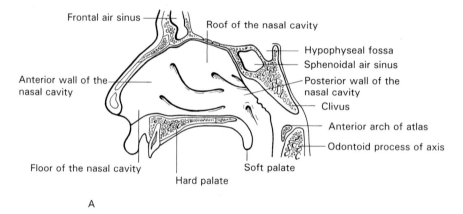

A

Fig. 1.2A
Sagittal section to show the shape of the nasal cavity.

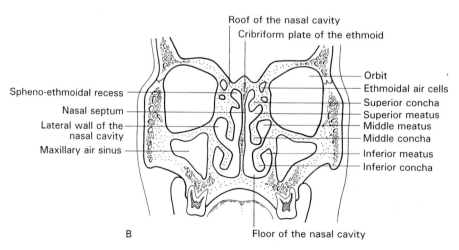

B

Fig. 1.2B
Coronal section to show the shape of the nasal cavity.

horizontally and the posterior third slopes posteriorly and inferiorly. The anterior one-third slopes down towards the tip of the nose. The middle one-third of the roof is virtually horizontal and runs parallel to the floor for a short distance. This part of the roof is formed from the cribriform plate of the ethmoid bone and houses the olfactory epithelium. The olfactory nerves perforate the cribriform plate to gain access to the olfactory bulb in the anterior cranial fossa. The posterior third of the roof is formed from the sphenoid and occipital bones (clivus) with the atlanto-occipital joint and the anterior arch of the atlas lying in close proximity. The sphenoidal air sinuses lie above the posterior third of the roof and directly above is the hypophyseal fossa for the pituitary gland.

The **floor** of the nasal cavity is horizontal and formed in front by the palatine process of the maxilla and behind by the horizontal plate of the palatine bone from which the soft palate is suspended.

The surface area of the **lateral wall** of the nose is greatly increased by the presence of 3 scrolls of bone (conchae or turbinates) that are covered with a thick and highly vascular mucoperiosteum (Fig. 1.3). The superior and middle conchae are part of the ethmoid bone whilst the inferior concha is a separate bone. Beneath the overhang of each concha is a recess in the lateral wall known as a meatus. The 3 conchae therefore separate the lateral wall into 4 areas: the 3 meatuses and a small area above the superior concha known as the spheno-ethmoidal recess, which receives the openings of the sphenoidal air cells. The superior meatus receives the openings of the posterior ethmoidal air cells, whilst the middle meatus receives the openings of the middle and anterior ethmoidal air cells and the maxillary and frontal air sinuses (Fig. 1.4). A bulge in the middle meatus, the bulla ethmoidalis, marks the location of the middle ethmoidal air cells, whilst the hiatus semilunaris, the groove directly below it, acts as a channel or gutter to direct the flow of secretions. The inferior meatus receives the nasolacrimal duct which drains tears from the medial corner of the eye. At the junction between the roof and lateral wall of the nose is the sphenopalatine foramen, through which vessels and nerves pass from the pterygopalatine fossa.

The **medial wall**, which is common to the two halves of the nasal cavity, is formed from the septal cartilage anteriorly and the vomer and perpendicular plate of the ethmoid posteriorly (Fig. 1.5).

The **internal nares** or choanae are separated from each other by the posterior margin of the vomer. They are bounded below by the horizontal plate of the palatine bone, above by the sphenoid bone and laterally by the medial pterygoid plate. The choanae represent the demarcation between the nasal cavity anteriorly and the commencement of the nasopharynx posteriorly.

Vascular supply of the nose

The arterial supply to the external nose arises through the facial artery as it passes across the face to the median palpebral fissure and sends lateral branches to supply the side of the nose, where it anastomoses with its partner from the opposite side. In addition, the external nose receives septal and alar branches from the superior labial artery, a lateral nasal branch from the facial artery, a dorsal nasal branch from the ophthalmic artery and a nasal branch from the infra-orbital branch of the maxillary artery.

The mucosa of the nasal cavity derives its arterial supply from the anterior and posterior ethmoidal branches of the ophthalmic artery, which supplies the

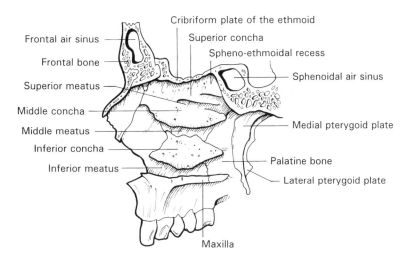

Fig. 1.3
The lateral wall of the nose.

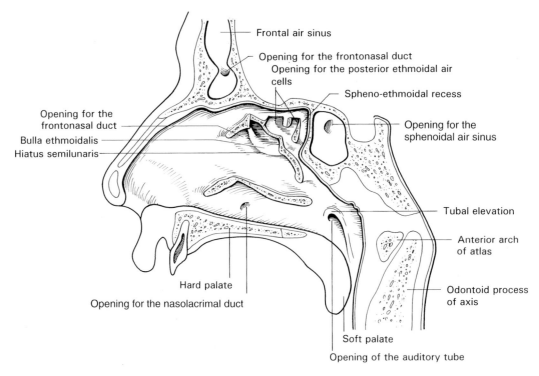

Fig. 1.4
The lateral wall of the nose with the conchae removed.

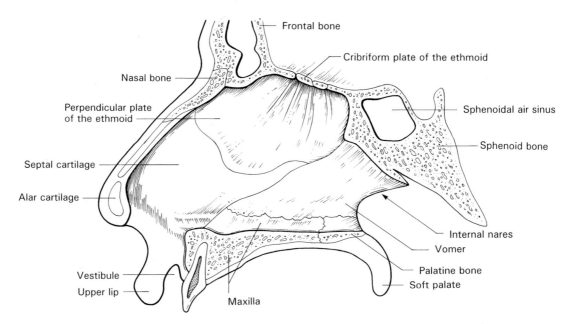

Fig. 1.5
The nasal septum.

roof of the cavity. The anterior ethmoidal artery also supplies the frontal and ethmoidal paranasal air sinuses, whilst the posterior ethmoidal artery supplies the ethmoidal and sphenoidal air sinuses. The anterior part of the nasal septum, conchae and meatuses derive their arterial supply from the sphenopalatine branch of the maxillary artery, which also supplies the ethmoidal air sinuses and anastomoses with the septal branch of the superior labial artery. This anastomosis is an important site of epistaxis within the vestibule.

The greater palatine artery also contributes to the arterial supply of the nasal cavity as, along with the facial and infra-orbital arteries, it supplies the maxillary air sinus.

Lymphatic drainage of the nose

The submandibular group of lymph nodes drains both the external nose and the nasal cavity, although the latter can also drain directly into the upper deep cervical group of nodes or via the retropharyngeal nodes. The lymphatic drainage of the frontal, anterior and middle ethmoidal and maxillary air sinuses is also into the submandibular nodes, whilst the posterior ethmoidal and sphenoidal sinuses drain into the retropharyngeal group.

SOMATIC INNERVATION OF THE NOSE

External nose

Sensory	Trigeminal (V^1) via anterior ethmoidal and external nasal branches of nasociliary nerve to bridge and tip of nose
	Trigeminal (V^2) via nasal branches from infra-orbital nerve to remainder of nose
Motor	Facial (VII) branches to muscles of facial expression

Nasal cavities (Figs 1.6 and 1.7)

Vestibule

Sensory	Trigeminal (V^1) via external nasal branches
	Trigeminal (V^2) via infra-orbital branch

Septum

Sensory	Trigeminal (V^1) via anterior ethmoidal branch to anterior and superior region
	Trigeminal (V^2) via nasopalatine branch from pterygopalatine ganglion to posterior and inferior region

Lateral wall and floor

Sensory	Trigeminal (V^1) via anterior ethmoidal branch to anterior and superior region
	Trigeminal (V^2) via anterior superior alveolar branch to anterior and inferior region
	Trigeminal (V^2) via posterior and inferior nasal branches from pterygopalatine ganglion to posterior and superior region
	Trigeminal (V^2) via greater palatine nerves from pterygopalatine ganglion to posterior and inferior region

Roof

Sensory	Olfactory (I) – special sensation of smell
	Trigeminal (V^1) via anterior ethmoidal nerve

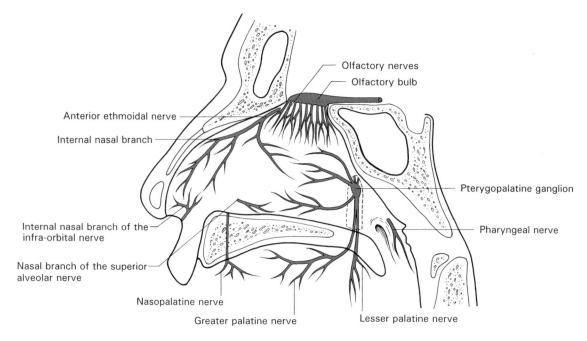

Fig. 1.6
The nerve supply of the lateral wall of the nose.

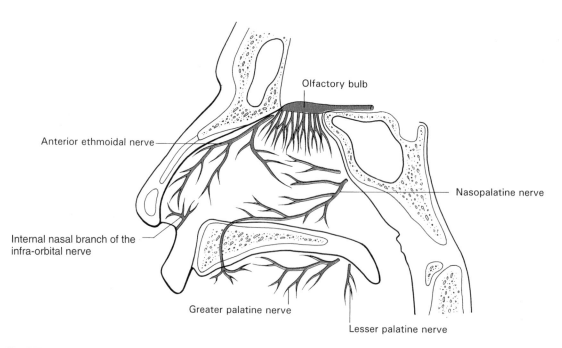

Fig. 1.7
The nerve supply of the medial wall of the nose.

THE ORAL CAVITY

The oral cavity extends between the lips anteriorly and the opening into the oropharynx posteriorly (Fig. 1.8). When the maxillary and mandibular dentition are brought into occlusion, the cavity is then separated into 2 quite distinct regions of unequal size – a smaller vestibule anteriorly and a larger oral cavity proper posteriorly. The 2 areas become continuous behind the last molar teeth.

The **vestibule** is a slit-like cavity bounded in front by the lips and cheeks and behind by the teeth and gums of both dental arcades. A small papilla is present on the mucous membrane of the cheek at the level of the upper second molar tooth, indicating the opening of the duct of the parotid salivary gland.

The oral cavity proper extends from the posterior surface of the dental arcades anteriorly to the isthmus of the fauces posteriorly. This opening into the oropharynx is bounded by the palatoglossal folds anteriorly and the palatopharyngeal folds posteriorly, with the palatine tonsils intervening between the two folds (Fig. 1.9).

The roof of the cavity is the **hard palate**, which is formed from the palatine process of the maxilla anteriorly and the horizontal plate of the palatine bone posteriorly. The anterior region of the hard palate also forms the floor of the nasal cavity. The oral surface of the palate is covered by a mucous membrane, which is tightly bound to the underlying periosteum and termed the mucoperiosteum.

The **soft palate** is suspended from the posterior surface of the hard palate and acts as a curtain between the nasal and oral regions of the pharynx. It has a free border which projects downwards into a midline uvula. The soft palate is considered in greater detail with the pharynx on page 11.

The floor of the oral cavity is formed largely by the root of the tongue and the reflection of mucous membrane from the sides of the tongue to the gum on the mandible. In the midline, a fold of mucous membrane (frenulum) connects the undersurface of the tongue to the floor of the mouth. On each side of the frenulum there is a small papilla, on the summit of which is the orifice of the duct of the submandibular

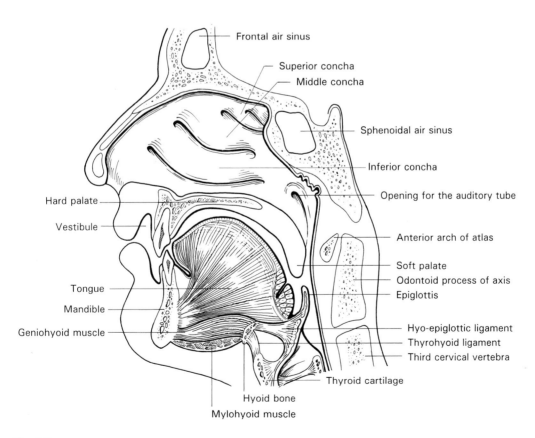

Frontal air sinus
Superior concha
Middle concha
Sphenoidal air sinus
Inferior concha
Opening for the auditory tube
Hard palate
Vestibule
Anterior arch of atlas
Soft palate
Odontoid process of axis
Epiglottis
Tongue
Mandible
Geniohyoid muscle
Hyo-epiglottic ligament
Thyrohyoid ligament
Third cervical vertebra
Thyroid cartilage
Hyoid bone
Mylohyoid muscle

Fig. 1.8
Sagittal section through the head.

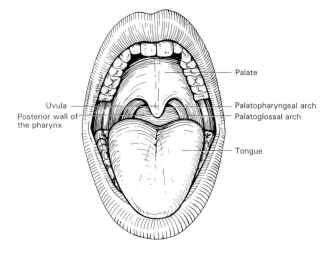

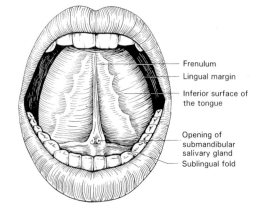

Fig. 1.9
Mouth open with tongue protracted.

Fig. 1.10
Mouth open with tongue elevated.

salivary gland (Fig. 1.10). From the papilla, a rounded ridge of mucous membrane (the sublingual fold) extends backwards and laterally, formed by the underlying sublingual salivary gland. Support of the mucosa and the root of the tongue is provided by the two mylohyoid muscles which stretch like a diaphragm from their origin along the mylohyoid line on the medial aspect of the body of the mandible on

each side, to their insertion along a median raphe and into the hyoid bone (Fig. 1.11).

Vascular supply of the oral cavity

The vestibule of the mouth receives its arterial supply from the superior and inferior labial branches of the facial artery. The upper teeth and supporting

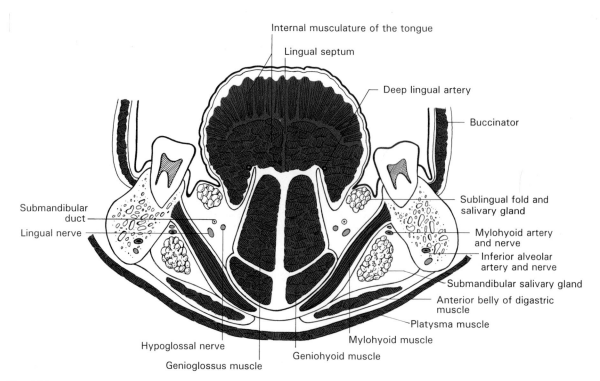

Fig. 1.11
Coronal section through the oral cavity.

structures are supplied by the superior alveolar arteries of the maxillary artery, and the lower teeth and supporting structures by the inferior alveolar artery, which also arises from the maxillary artery. The principal artery to the tongue and floor of the mouth is the lingual artery, supported by the tonsillar and ascending palatine branches of the facial artery. The palate derives its arterial supply from the greater palatine branch of the maxillary artery, the ascending palatine branch of the facial artery and the palatine branch of the ascending pharyngeal artery.

Lymphatic drainage of the oral cavity

The teeth and gums of the upper jaw drain into the submandibular nodes and then to the subclavicular group, whilst the lower teeth and supporting structures drain to the submental nodes and then to the paratracheal group. The lymphatic drainage of the hard palate is via the upper deep cervical group, whilst the soft palate drains to both the retromandibular and upper deep cervical group. The floor of the mouth and tongue have a complicated pattern of lymphatic drainage to the submental, submandibular, jugulodigastric, jugulo-omohyoid and deep cervical groups. The lymphatic drainage of the palatine tonsils is to the jugulodigastric nodes.

SOMATIC INNERVATION OF THE ORAL CAVITY
(Figs 1.12 and 1.13)

Vestibule

Sensory	Trigeminal (V^2 and V^3) via alveolar and labial branches
Motor	Facial (VII)

Hard palate

Sensory	Trigeminal (V^2) via palatine and nasopalatine branches
Taste	Facial (VII) via branches of V^2

Soft palate

Sensory	Trigeminal (V^2) via palatine branches to anterior region. Glossopharyngeal (IX) to posterior region
Motor	Trigeminal (V^3) to tensor veli palatini Via pharyngeal plexus (IX, X and XI) to all other muscles
Taste	Facial (VII) via greater petrosal nerve

Tongue

Sensory	Trigeminal (V^3) via lingual nerve to anterior 2/3 Glossopharyngeal (IX) to posterior 2/3
Motor	Pharyngeal plexus (IX, X & XI) to palatoglossus Hypoglossal (XII) to all other muscles
Taste	Facial (VII) via chorda tympani to anterior 2/3 Glossopharyngeal (IX) to posterior 2/3

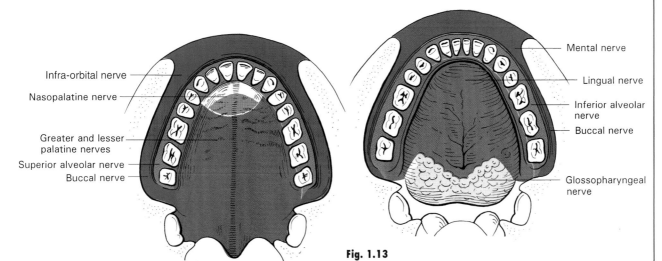

Fig. 1.12
Sensory innervation of the palate and upper dentition.

Fig. 1.13
Sensory innervation of the floor of the mouth and lower dentition.

10 THE PHARYNX

The pharynx is a midline, funnel-shaped, longitudinal, muscular tube whose dual function is to convey air to and from the larynx and ingested food to the esophagus (Fig. 1.14). It extends from the base of the skull above, passes down behind the nose, mouth and larynx and becomes continuous with the esophagus at the level of the sixth cervical vertebra. The roof of the pharynx is limited above by the body of the sphenoid and the basilar region of the occipital bones. The posterior wall is separated from the anterior surfaces of the bodies of the upper 6 cervical vertebrae by the retropharyngeal space and prevertebral fascia, which permits free movement during deglutition and phonation. The anterior wall is deficient, with openings into the nasal cavity, oral cavity and larynx (Fig. 1.15).

The pharyngeal wall is composed of 4 layers. These are (from internal to external):

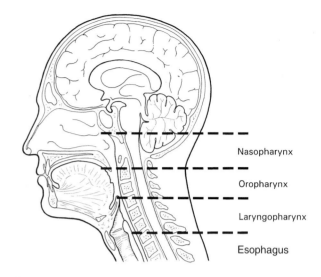

Nasopharynx

Oropharynx

Laryngopharynx

Esophagus

Fig. 1.14
The divisions of the pharynx.

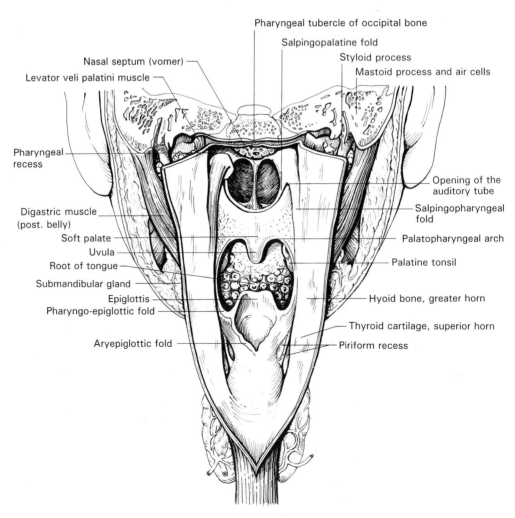

Pharyngeal tubercle of occipital bone

Salpingopalatine fold

Styloid process

Mastoid process and air cells

Nasal septum (vomer)

Levator veli palatini muscle

Pharyngeal recess

Digastric muscle (post. belly)

Soft palate

Uvula

Root of tongue

Submandibular gland

Epiglottis

Pharyngo-epiglottic fold

Aryepiglottic fold

Opening of the auditory tube

Salpingopharyngeal fold

Palatopharyngeal arch

Palatine tonsil

Hyoid bone, greater horn

Thyroid cartilage, superior horn

Piriform recess

Fig. 1.15
Dorsal view of the pharynx.

1. a mucous membrane that is continuous with all structures that open into the pharynx
2. a submucosa comprising a tough fibrous pharyngobasilar fascia that is firmly attached to the base of the skull and gives a rigidity only found in the upper region of the pharynx
3. a muscular layer
4. loose connective tissue forming the buccopharyngeal fascia.

The pharynx is topographically and functionally separated into thirds – an upper nasopharynx, a middle oropharynx and a lower laryngopharynx.

The **nasopharynx** is continuous with the nasal cavity anteriorly and with the oropharynx inferiorly, via the pharyngeal isthmus, and therefore lies behind the nose and above the soft palate. It is solely respiratory in function and is lined with ciliated columnar epithelium. Due to the thickness of the pharyngobasilar fascia in this region, the walls are relatively rigid and patent at all times, thereby presenting no obstruction to respiration. The space is best described as having anterior limits, a sloping roof, a posterior wall, lateral walls and a floor.

The anterior limits of the nasopharynx are the internal nares and the posterior border of the nasal septum. The roof and posterior wall abut against the basilar part of the occipital bone, the anterior arch of the atlas and the body of the axis respectively. In the mucosa of the upper end of the posterior wall is the pharyngeal tonsil (adenoids when enlarged). The

lateral wall houses the opening of the pharyngotympanic (auditory or Eustachian) tube which communicates with the cavity of the middle ear (Fig. 1.16). The opening is directed downwards, with a hood-like overhang formed by the medial end of the tubal cartilage. The groove behind the opening is the pharyngeal recess. The salpingopharyngeal fold stretches downwards from the tubal elevation and contains the salpingopharyngeus muscle (p. 14). Contraction of this muscle during swallowing opens the auditory aditus and thus equalizes air pressure on either side of the tympanic membrane. The tubal tonsils are lymphoid tissue found in close proximity to the auditory opening.

The floor of the nasopharynx is formed by the soft palate, and when this is elevated it closes off the nasopharynx from the oropharynx. The gap between the posterior free margin of the soft palate and the posterior wall of the pharynx is the pharyngeal isthmus.

The **soft palate** is suspended from the posterior border of the palatine bone and acts as a movable curtain separating the nasopharynx from the oropharynx. During normal respiration, when it is relaxed, the soft palate hangs down into the oropharynx and thus the airway remains patent. The soft palate is elevated only during phonation and deglutition, and therefore this is the only time when the oropharynx is truly demarcated from the nasopharynx.

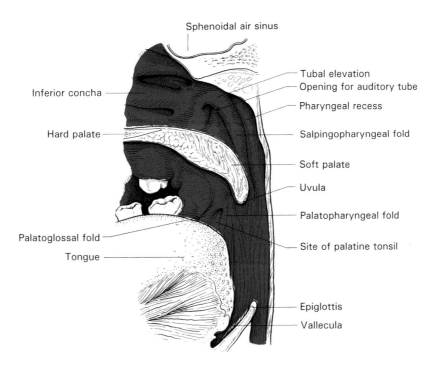

Fig. 1.16
The lateral wall of the nasopharynx.

The soft palate consists of a fold of mucous membrane enclosing the central aponeurosis of the tensor veli palatini muscles to which all other muscles of the soft palate are attached (Fig. 1.17). The mucous membrane on the nasal surface of the soft palate is respiratory in nature, whilst that covering the oral surface is gustatory. The anterior border of the soft palate is firmly attached to the posterior margin of the hard palate, whilst the posterior border and the midline uvula hang free. The lateral borders are connected to the tongue by the palatoglossal mucosal folds and to the pharynx by the palatopharyngeal mucosal folds.

The soft palate is elevated to close off the nasopharynx during swallowing, sucking, speech and blowing, and can also change shape, so helping to guide the bolus of food through the oropharyngeal isthmus. On elevation, the soft palate is pulled upwards and backwards and the uvula helps to further close off the pharyngeal isthmus.

The muscles associated with the soft palate are the levator veli palatini, tensor veli palatini, palatoglossus, palatopharyngeus and musculus uvulae (Table 1.1). All are innervated by the pharyngeal plexus with the exception of the tensor that is supplied by the mandibular division of the trigeminal nerve (Figs 1.17 and 1.18).

The **oropharynx** connects the nasopharynx above to the laryngopharynx below and opens anteriorly into the oral cavity via the oropharyngeal isthmus. This is

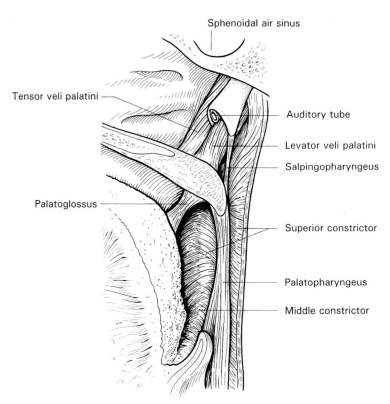

Fig. 1.17
The muscles of the soft palate and upper pharynx.

Table 1.1
Muscles of the soft palate

	Origin	Insertion
Tensor veli palatini	Spine of sphenoid, auditory tube, scaphoid fossa	Forms palatine aponeurosis
Levator veli palatini	Petrous temporal bone, auditory tube	Upper surface of palatine aponeurosis
Palatoglossus	Undersurface of palatine aponeurosis	Side of tongue
Palatopharyngeus	Posterior border of hard palate, palatine aponeurosis	Posterior border of lamina of thyroid cartilage
Musculus uvulae	Posterior border of hard palate, palatine aponeurosis	Mucous membrane of uvula

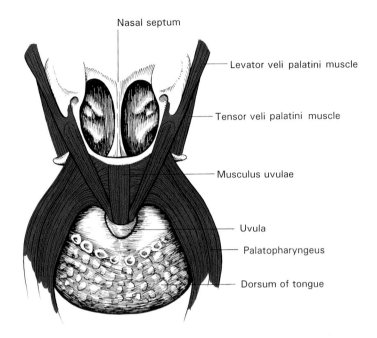

Fig. 1.18
The muscles of the soft palate as seen from behind.

formed anteriorly from the palatoglossal folds and posteriorly from the palatopharyngeal folds, which are folds of mucous membrane that cover the muscles of the same name. Between the two folds are the palatine tonsils, sitting in a recess called the tonsillar sinus. These tonsils may extend upwards into the soft palate and medially into the tongue. The pharyngeal, palatine and lingual tonsils form an incomplete circle of lymphoid tissue around the superior part of the pharynx which is called the tonsillar ring (Waldeyer's ring). The roof of the oropharynx is formed from the lower surface of the soft palate and its inferior boundary is the dorsal third of the tongue and the superior border of the epiglottis. Its posterior wall is formed from the constrictor muscles lying in close proximity to the second and third cervical vertebrae. The oropharynx is lined with stratified squamous epithelium indicating its gustatory function despite being a common passage for the respiratory system.

The **laryngopharynx** extends from the superior border of the epiglottis above to the lower border of the cricoid cartilage below. The posterior wall is formed from the middle and inferior constrictor muscles and the stylopharyngeus and palatopharyngeus muscles. The posterior wall extends from the lower border of the second cervical vertebra above to the upper border of the sixth cervical vertebra below, where the laryngopharynx becomes continuous with the esophagus.

The laryngopharynx opens anteriorly into the larynx and its boundaries are therefore the laryngeal inlet

with the aryepiglottic folds above and the posterior borders of the arytenoid and cricoid cartilages below. The laryngeal inlet bulges into the laryngopharynx leaving two hollows, one on either side, called the piriform recess fossa, which is bounded by an aryepiglottic fold medially and the thyroid cartilage and thyrohyoid membrane laterally. Deep to the mucous membrane of the piriform recess are the internal and inferior laryngeal nerves.

The upper region of the laryngopharynx has a dual function – the passage of both air and food – and must therefore remain patent at all times. The lower region is, however, solely associated with the alimentary system and so the walls are opposed and continuous with the esophagus.

Muscles of the pharynx

There are 2 distinct muscle groups associated with the pharynx – an outer circular layer whose function is to constrict the pharynx and an inner longitudinal layer whose function is to elevate the pharynx (Fig. 1.19, Table 1.2)

The constrictors of the pharynx are paired muscles that interdigitate in a posterior midline raphe (Fig. 1.20). There are 3 constrictors – superior, middle and inferior, which form the greater part of the lateral and posterior walls of the pharynx. The arrangement of the constrictors is such that, when viewed from the outside, they fit one inside each other like stacking

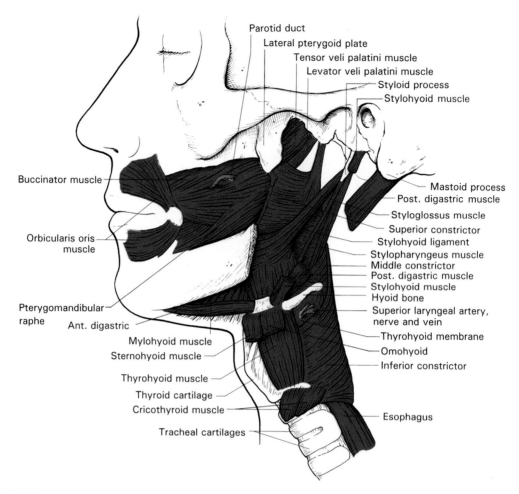

Fig. 1.19
Lateral view of the oropharyngeal muscles.

Table 1.2
Muscles of the pharynx

	Origin	Insertion
Superior constrictor	Medial pterygoid plate, pterygoid hamulus, pterygomandibular ligament, mylohyoid line	Pharyngeal tubercle, median fibrous raphe
Middle constrictor	Stylohyoid ligament, greater and lesser horns of hyoid bone	Median fibrous raphe
Inferior constrictor	Oblique line on thyroid cartilage, side of cricoid cartilage	Median fibrous raphe
Stylopharyngeus	Styloid process	Posterior border of thyroid cartilage
Salpingopharyngeus	Auditory tube	Blends with palatopharyngeus
Palatopharyngeus	Posterior border of hard palate, palatine aponeurosis	Posterior border of lamina of thyroid cartilage

flower pots, thereby forming an overlapping and virtually continuous muscular tube.

The elevators of the pharynx operate during swallowing and phonation and form the inner longitudinal muscular layer of the pharynx. The most posterior of the muscles arises from the styloid process,

the middle one from the region of the auditory tube and the most anterior from the posterior border of the hard palate.

The space between the skull and superior constrictor is the gateway to the nasopharynx, and the levators veli palatini, auditory tubes and the ascending palatine

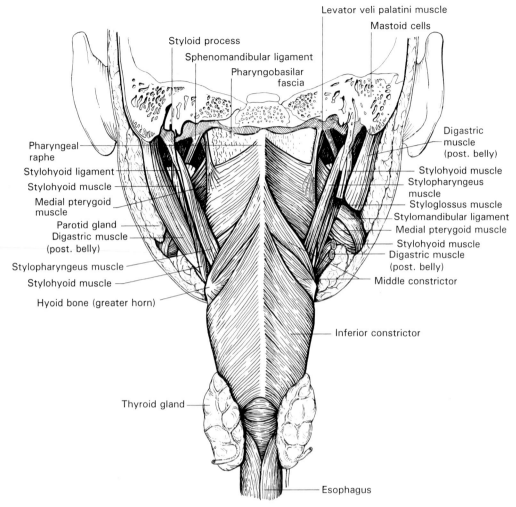

Fig. 1.20
Dorsal view of the pharyngeal muscles.

arteries gain entry via this route. The space between the superior and middle constrictors is the gateway to the mouth, through which the stylopharyngeus muscles, the glossopharyngeal nerves and the stylohyoid ligaments pass. The space between the middle and inferior constrictors is the gateway to the larynx, through which the internal laryngeal nerves and superior laryngeal arteries and veins pass.

The recurrent laryngeal nerve and the inferior laryngeal artery pierce the pharyngeal wall below the level of the inferior constrictor. The inferior constrictor muscle is sometimes described as being in two parts – the thyropharyngeus superiorly and the cricopharyngeus inferiorly, with the dehiscence of Killian between, which is a site of potential herniation.

Deglutition (swallowing)

Deglutition consists of 3 distinct phases: the first is voluntary, whilst the others are essentially involuntary:

Phase 1 – Following mastication, the bolus of food is pushed towards the oropharynx by the action of the intrinsic muscles of the tongue against the hard palate.

Phase 2 – Respiration is temporarily halted during this phase, which is involuntary and is initiated when the food reaches the oropharyngeal isthmus. The opening back into the oral cavity is closed off by the contraction of the palatoglossal muscles and the food is propelled into the oropharynx. It is at this stage that the oral cavity and oropharynx become isolated from the nasopharynx and larynx. The soft palate is tensed by the tensor veli palatini and raised by the levator veli palatini to shut off the nasopharynx, and contraction of the superior constrictor ensures a tight seal. The laryngeal opening is constricted by the aryepiglottic folds and the transverse arytenoid muscles, and the larynx is pulled forward by the action of the suprahyoid muscles on the hyoid bone. The larynx is then elevated by the action of the longitudinal muscles of the pharynx which approximates the larynx to the dorsum of the tongue and allows the epiglottis to act in a protective role to prevent food from entering the laryngeal opening. The salpingopharyngeus muscle also contracts at this stage and, because of its attachment to the auditory tube, equalizes the pressure on both sides of the tympanic membrane. The bolus passes over the epiglottis, or if more liquid runs in the piriform recesses, and into the laryngopharynx. Its passage from the oropharynx to the esophagus is controlled by the consecutive contraction of the constrictor muscles.

Phase 3 – Once food is present in the esophagus, peristaltic waves ensure its progression down into the stomach. As the food enters the esophagus the hyoid bone and laryngeal cartilages return to their resting position and the soft palate is relaxed.

The **innervation of deglutition** is complex but can be simplified as follows:

Stage 1 is controlled by the somatic (tongue) muscles assisted by the external branchial muscles such as the mylohyoid, stylohyoid and digastric, influencing the hyoid bone and the floor of the mouth.

Stage 2 is controlled by internal branchial muscles such as palatopharyngeus, stylopharyngeus and the constrictors.

Stage 3 is taken over by the involuntary striated and smooth muscles of the upper and lower esophagus respectively, the nerve supply of which passes from branchial efferent to visceral efferent.

Thus, during deglutition there is a gradual transfer of nervous control from somatic efferent → external branchial efferent (voluntary) → internal branchial efferent (involuntary) → visceral efferent (involuntary).

Vascular supply of the pharynx

The blood supply of the pharynx is derived from the ascending pharyngeal artery, ascending palatine and tonsillar branches of the facial artery, the greater palatine, pharyngeal and pterygoid branches of the maxillary artery and pharyngeal branches from the superior and inferior thyroid arteries. The region of the epiglottis derives its arterial supply from the dorsal lingual artery, which is a branch of the lingual artery.

Lymphatic drainage of the pharynx

The lymphatic drainage of the pharynx passes to the deep cervical group of lymph nodes either directly or via the retropharyngeal or paratracheal group of nodes. The lymphatic drainage of the epiglottis passes to the infrahyoid group of nodes.

Innervation of the pharynx

The principal innervation of the pharynx is via the pharyngeal plexus (Figs 1.21 and 1.22) which is formed

on the external surface of the middle constrictor muscle, opposite the greater horn of the hyoid bone. It arises from pharyngeal branches of cranial nerves IX, X and XI along with branches from the superior cervical sympathetic ganglion. From this plexus, branches penetrate into the substance of the pharynx and are responsible for much of the innervation to this region. The glossopharyngeal (IX) nerve is the principal sensory nerve, whilst the cranial part of the accessory (XI) via the vagus (X) is the main motor supply. The sympathetic component is largely vasomotor is nature.

SOMATIC INNERVATION OF THE PHARYNX

Nasopharynx

Sensory	Trigeminal (V²) via pterygopalatine ganglion
	Glossopharyngeal (IX) to lower regions

Oropharynx

Sensory	Glossopharyngeal (IX)
Taste	Glossopharyngeal (IX) to region of palatoglossal arch and oropharynx
	Facial (VII) and glossopharyngeal (IX) to soft palate
	Vagus (X) via branch of superior laryngeal nerve to region of epiglottis

Laryngopharynx

Sensory	Glossopharyngeal (IX)

Motor innervation

Pharyngeal plexus to all muscles of pharynx and soft palate except:

Stylopharyngeus via glossopharyngeal (IX)

Tensor veli palatini via trigeminal (V³)

THE LARYNX

The larynx is the first part of the lower respiratory tract and is formed from a complex arrangement of cartilages, muscles, ligaments and membranes. It is a midline structure which extends between the third and sixth cervical vertebrae in the adult, although in the infant it may only extend as far as the inferior border of the fourth cervical vertebra. It is superficial and readily palpated, as it is covered only by skin, the platysma muscle and superficial and deep layers of fascia.

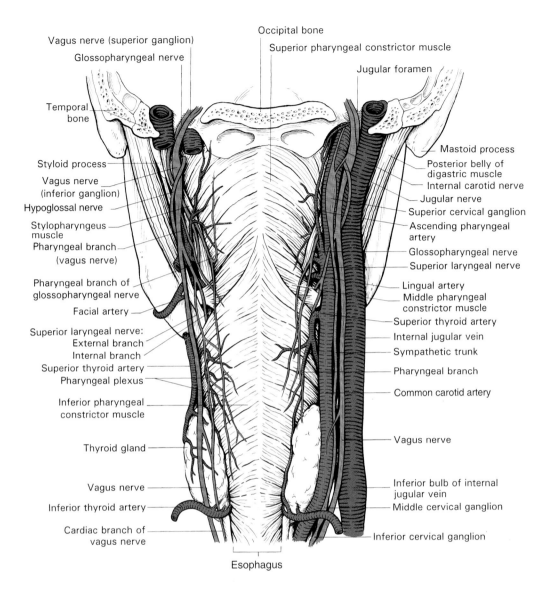

Fig. 1.21
Nerves and vessels on the dorsal and lateral walls of the pharynx.

Posteriorly it is separated from the cervical column by the pharynx and thin prevertebral muscles. It communicates with the laryngopharynx behind and with the trachea below. Its rigid skeletal structure ensures that it remains patent at all times, which is essential for its primary role as a respiratory passage. It has also developed a protective valve mechanism at the inlet to prevent entry of foreign material from the laryngopharynx.

Given the complex function of the larynx it is not surprising that its anatomy is somewhat intricate and highly specialized. The larynx has had to compromise between the need for rigidity for its respiratory

purpose and the need for mobility to fulfil its function as a valve and mechanism for phonation.

Although the **hyoid bone** is not an intrinsic part of the larynx, it is firmly attached to the laryngeal cartilages, and movement of the hyoid is accompanied by the concomitant movement of the larynx. The larynx itself is formed from 9 cartilages, 3 of which are midline and singular and 6 of which are paired and more laterally placed (Fig. 1.23). The 3 midline cartilages are the epiglottis (elastic), the thyroid (hyaline) and the cricoid (hyaline), and the 3 more lateral pairs are the arytenoids (hyaline and elastic), the cuneiforms (elastic) and the corniculate cartilages (elastic)

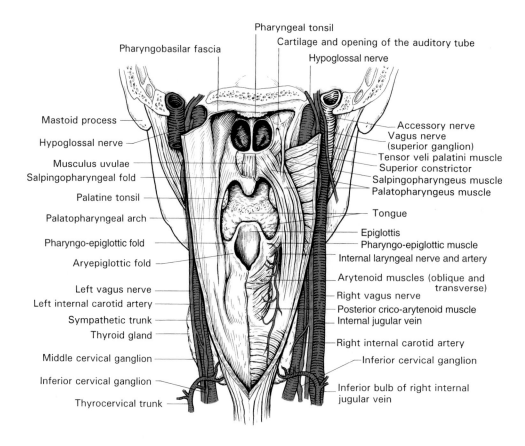

Fig. 1.22
View of the pharynx with the posterior aspect of the constrictors opened.

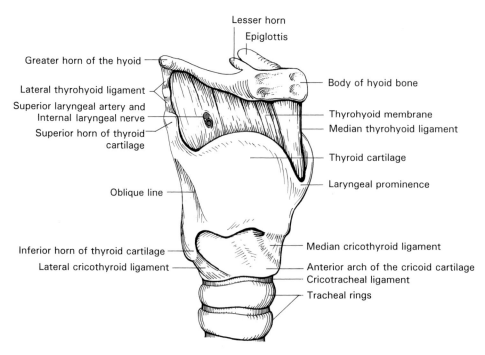

Fig. 1.23
Lateral view of the hyoid bone and laryngeal skeleton.

(Fig. 1.24). Of the paired cartilages, the arytenoids are arguably the most important. Those cartilages that are hyaline in form, namely the thyroid, cricoid and basal parts of the arytenoids, may undergo ossification with advancing age. Although complete ossification of the cartilages is rare until old age, ossification may in fact commence as early as 18 years of age.

The **thyroid cartilage** is the largest of the laryngeal cartilages, and is a midline structure composed of 2 quadrilateral laminae fused anteriorly in the midline to form the laryngeal prominence. The posterior border of each lamine is free and receives fibers of the stylopharyngeus and palatopharyngeus muscles. This border is extended upwards to form the superior horn and downwards to form the inferior horn. The superior border of the thyroid cartilage is connected to the superior border of the hyoid bone by the fibrous thyrohyoid membrane, which is pierced laterally by the internal laryngeal nerve and the superior laryngeal artery. The membrane is thickened in the midline to form the median thyrohyoid ligament and laterally, at its free border, to form the lateral thyrohyoid ligaments. These lateral ligaments connect the superior horns of the thyroid cartilage to the hyoid bone and may contain small grain-like nodules of cartilage (cartilago triticea).

The inferior horn of the thyroid articulates via synovial joints with the cricoid cartilage below. Movement at these facets allows the thyroid to tilt or glide on the cricoid rather as a visor moves on a crash helmet.

The external surface of each lamina has an oblique line for the attachment of the sternothyroid, thyrohyoid and inferior constrictor muscles. The internal surface of each thyroid lamina is smooth and covered by mucous membrane. Attached anteriorly to the posterior surface of the thyroid cartilage are the stem of the epiglottis, the vocal and vestibular ligaments and the thyroarytenoid, thyroepiglottic and vocalis muscles.

The **cricoid cartilage** is smaller than the thyroid but is thicker, stronger and more fixed in position. It lies at the level of the sixth cervical vertebra and is the only completely rigid region of the larynx. It articulates with the thyroid cartilage above and is connected below to the first tracheal ring via the cricotracheal membrane. It is shaped like a signet ring, with a broad posterior lamina and a narrower anterior arch. The lamina has a midline ridge for the attachment of muscle fibers of the esophagus and 2 lateral hollows that are the site of attachment of the posterior cricoarytenoid muscles. The cricothyroid and inferior constrictor muscles take their origin from the arch, which is also the location of the articular facets for the thyroid cartilage. The upper border of the cricoid cartilage is connected to the thyroid cartilage by the cricothyroid membrane which is also known as the conus elasticus and forms part of the important fibro-elastic membrane of the larynx. Although the superior border of the cricothyroid membrane is free, it is attached anteriorly to the posterior surface of the thyroid cartilage and posteriorly to the vocal process of the arytenoid

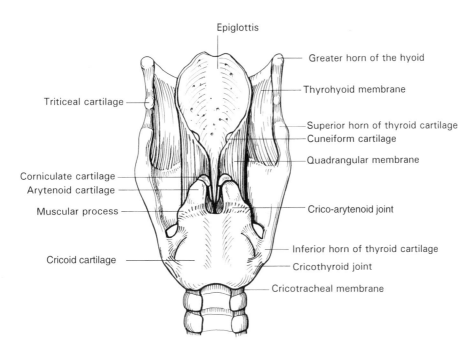

Fig. 1.24
Posterior view of the laryngeal skeleton.

Epiglottis

Greater horn of the hyoid

Thyrohyoid membrane

Superior horn of thyroid cartilage

Cuneiform cartilage

Quadrangular membrane

Triticeal cartilage

Corniculate cartilage

Arytenoid cartilage

Muscular process

Crico-arytenoid joint

Cricoid cartilage

Inferior horn of thyroid cartilage

Cricothyroid joint

Cricotracheal membrane

cartilages. This is known as the vocal fold and the space between the membrane of each side is the rima glottidis. The median portion of the cricothyroid membrane is thickened to form the cricothyroid ligament. The superior border of the cartilage offers attachment for the lateral cricoarytenoid muscles and is the location of the synovial articular facets for the arytenoid cartilages.

Laryngotomy is usually undertaken as an emergency procedure for the relief of acute airway obstruction. An incision is made in the relatively bloodless field immediately above the cricoid cartilage, and the skin, subcutaneous tissues and the cricothyroid membrane are punctured with a single stab incision (Fig. 1.25 A–B).

The **arytenoid cartilages** are shaped like three-sided pyramids, with an inferior base that articulates with the superior border of the cricoid cartilage, an anterior vocal process, a lateral muscular process and a superior apex (Fig. 1.26). The vocal ligament of the cricothyroid membrane attaches to the vocal process, and the posterior and lateral cricoarytenoid muscles attach to the muscular process. The small corniculate cartilages are found at the apex of the arytenoid cartilage within the aryepiglottic fold. The posterior surfaces of the cartilages are united by the transverse arytenoid muscles, whilst the anterolateral surface of the cartilage

provides attachment for the thyroarytenoid and vocalis muscles. The quadrangular membrane is the second part of the fibro-elastic membrane of the larynx and it stretches between the arytenoid cartilages and the epiglottis. The anterior border of this membrane, which arises from the lower half of the epiglottis, is higher than its posterior border, which attaches to the vocal process of the arytenoid. Its superior border is sloped and forms the aryepiglottic folds which carry the cuneiform cartilages. During deglutition the laryngeal inlet is closed and the cuneiform cartilages become approximated to the tubercle of the epiglottis. The lower border of the quadrangular membrane is free and forms the vestibular ligament or false cord.

The **epiglottis** is shaped like a leaf or, perhaps more realistically, a bicycle seat. It stands vertically behind the hyoid bone and the root of the tongue and overhangs the laryngeal inlet. It is broad superiorly with a free border which tapers inferiorly to be attached to the inner surface of the thyroid cartilage by the thyroepiglottic ligament. The anterior surface of the epiglottis is attached to the hyoid bone via the hyo-epiglottic ligament. The mucous membrane covering this surface is reflected onto the root and sides of the tongue as one median and two lateral glosso-epiglottic folds, and the depressions that form between them are the valleculae. The posterior border is free, with an elevation in the lower part known as the epiglottic tubercle. The epiglottis is connected to the arytenoid cartilages via the aryepiglottic folds.

The **laryngeal cavity** is separated into 3 topographical regions:

1. an upper vestibule or supraglottic region which extends from the laryngeal inlet to the vestibular folds or cords
2. the ventricle or glottic region which extends between the vestibular and vocal folds

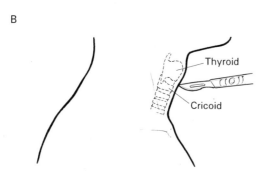

A

Body of hyoid bone

Greater horn of hyoid bone

Lateral lobe of thyroid gland

Thyroid cartilage

Cricothyroid membrane

Cricoid cartilage

Isthmus of thyroid gland

First tracheal ring

B

Thyroid

Cricoid

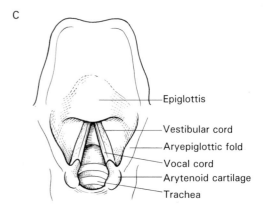

C

Epiglottis

Vestibular cord

Aryepiglottic fold

Vocal cord

Arytenoid cartilage

Trachea

Fig. 1.25
(A) Anterior aspect of the neck. (B) Lateral aspect of the neck showing site of laryngotomy.

(C) View of the larynx at laryngoscopy.

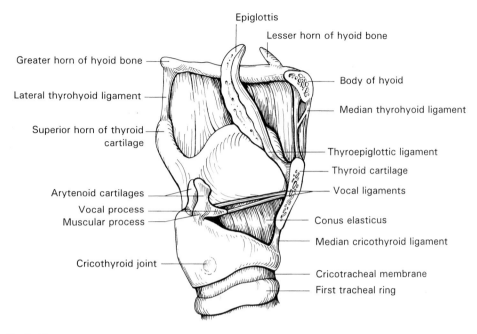

Epiglottis

Lesser horn of hyoid bone

Greater horn of hyoid bone

Lateral thyrohyoid ligament

Superior horn of thyroid cartilage

Arytenoid cartilages
Vocal process
Muscular process

Cricothyroid joint

Body of hyoid

Median thyrohyoid ligament

Thyroepiglottic ligament
Thyroid cartilage
Vocal ligaments

Conus elasticus

Median cricothyroid ligament

Cricotracheal membrane
First tracheal ring

Fig. 1.26
Lateral view of the larynx with the right half of the thyroid cartilage removed.

3. an infraglottic region which extends from below the vocal folds to the beginning of the trachea (Fig. 1.27).

The **laryngeal inlet** is the opening into the larynx from the laryngopharynx. It is bounded anteriorly by the upper edge of the epiglottis, posteriorly by a

membrane between the arytenoid cartilages, and laterally by the aryepiglottic folds containing the cuneiform and corniculate cartilages.

The lateral walls of the **vestibule** are formed from the quadrangular membrane and the medial surfaces of the aryepiglottic folds. Its superior boundary is the

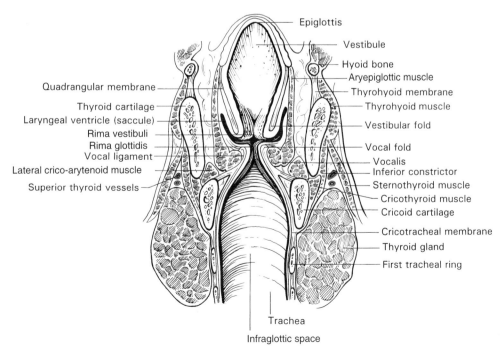

Epiglottis
Vestibule
Hyoid bone
Aryepiglottic muscle
Thyrohyoid membrane
Thyrohyoid muscle

Quadrangular membrane

Thyroid cartilage
Laryngeal ventricle (saccule)
Rima vestibuli
Rima glottidis
Vocal ligament
Lateral crico-arytenoid muscle
Superior thyroid vessels

Vestibular fold

Vocal fold
Vocalis
Inferior constrictor
Sternothyroid muscle
Cricothyroid muscle
Cricoid cartilage

Cricotracheal membrane
Thyroid gland
First tracheal ring

Trachea
Infraglottic space

Fig. 1.27
Coronal section through the larynx.

aryepiglottic folds and its inferior boundary is the vestibular ligaments (the free inferior border of the quadrangular membrane) which stretch between the arytenoid and thyroid cartilages. Its anterior wall is the sloping posterior surface of the epiglottis with its protruding tubercle; its posterior wall is short, being formed from the upper part of the arytenoid cartilages.

The **ventricle** is the smallest of the 3 regions of the larynx and is situated between the vestibular folds above and the vocal folds below. On each side it opens through a slit between the folds into a recess called the laryngeal sinus. From the anterior part of the sinus a narrow opening leads into the saccule of the larynx. There is a dense accumulation of mucous glands in the saccule that secrete mucous onto the vocal folds. The rima glottidis is the fissure that exists between the two vocal folds and stretches between the vocal processes of the arytenoid cartilages behind and the posterior surface of the thyroid cartilage in front. This is the narrowest part of the larynx and the most important in terms of phonation.

The **infraglottic** region has the lower part of the thyroid cartilage, the cricothyroid membrane and the arch of the cricoid cartilage as its anterior boundary, whilst the posterior boundary is formed from the lamina of the cricoid cartilage. The lateral walls are formed from the cricothyroid membrane (conus elasticus). The upper part is elliptical in shape but adopts a more circular outline as it approaches the trachea.

Muscles of the larynx

The muscles of the larynx (Table 1.3) are classified as either extrinsic or intrinsic with the former (inferior constrictor, all supra- and infrahyoid strap muscles) being responsible for moving the larynx as a whole in relation to other structures, while the latter are responsible for controlling the shape of the inlet and the position and tension of the vocal folds (Figs 1.28 and 1.29).

The **muscles of the inlet** have a sphincteric action and are responsible for closing the laryngeal inlet thereby acting in a protective capacity during swallowing. Contraction of the transverse and oblique arytenoids and the aryepiglottic muscles brings the aryepiglottic folds together and pulls the arytenoid cartilages toward the epiglottis (Fig. 1.30). The transverse arytenoid muscle passes from the posterior surface of one arytenoid cartilage to the posterior surface of the other, whilst the oblique arytenoids are more superficial and cross each other to become continuous as the aryepiglottic muscle in the aryepiglottic fold. The thyroepiglottic muscle arises from the internal surface of the thyroid lamina and inserts into the lateral margin of the epiglottis. The sphincteric action of the inlet only occurs during swallowing and plays no part in phonation, coughing, etc.

The **muscles of the vocal folds** work in opposing pairs and are responsible for either opening/closing or lengthening/shortening the vocal folds. The movements of opening and closing of the vocal folds take place at the crico-arytenoid joints. Opening (abduction) is effected by the posterior crico-arytenoid muscles that arise from the posterior lamina of the cricoid cartilage and insert into the muscular process of the arytenoid cartilages. Closing (adduction) of the vocal folds is effected by the lateral crico-arytenoids that arise from the arch of the cricoid cartilage and insert into the muscular process of the arytenoid cartilages. This action is reinforced by contraction of the transverse arytenoid muscles.

Table 1.3
Muscles of the larynx

	Origin	Insertion	Action
Cricothyroid	Side of cricoid cartilage	Inferior horn and margin of thyroid cartilage	Tenses vocal folds
Posterior crico-arytenoid	Posterior of lamina of cricoid cartilage	Muscular process of arytenoid cartilage	Abducts vocal folds
Lateral crico-arytenoid	Arch of cricoid cartilage	Muscular process of arytenoid cartilage	Adducts vocal folds
Thyro-arytenoid	Posterior surface of thyroid cartilage	Anterior lateral surface of arytenoid cartilage	Relaxes vocal folds
Transverse arytenoid	Posterior and medial surface of arytenoid cartilage	Posterior and medial surface of opposite arytenoid cartilage	Closes rima glottidis
Oblique arytenoid	Muscular process of arytenoid cartilage	Apex of opposite arytenoid cartilage	Closes rima glottidis
Vocalis	Angle between laminae of thyroid cartilage	Vocal process of arytenoid cartilage	Alters vocal folds

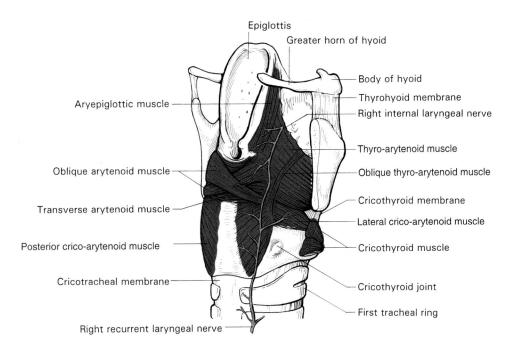

Epiglottis
Greater horn of hyoid
Body of hyoid
Thyrohyoid membrane
Right internal laryngeal nerve
Thyro-arytenoid muscle
Oblique thyro-arytenoid muscle
Cricothyroid membrane
Lateral crico-arytenoid muscle
Cricothyroid muscle
Cricothyroid joint
First tracheal ring
Aryepiglottic muscle
Oblique arytenoid muscle
Transverse arytenoid muscle
Posterior crico-arytenoid muscle
Cricotracheal membrane
Right recurrent laryngeal nerve

Fig. 1.28
The laryngeal musculature.

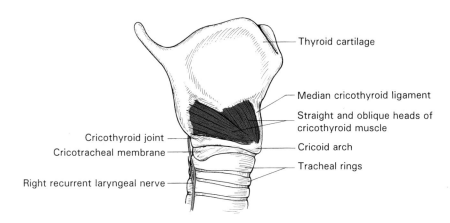

Thyroid cartilage
Median cricothyroid ligament
Straight and oblique heads of cricothyroid muscle
Cricoid arch
Tracheal rings
Cricothyroid joint
Cricotracheal membrane
Right recurrent laryngeal nerve

Fig. 1.29
Lateral view of the cricothyroid musculature.

Lengthening and shortening of the vocal folds takes place at the cricothyroid joints. Lengthening (tensing) of the vocal folds is brought about by the action of the cricothyroid muscle, which arises from the arch of the cricoid cartilage and inserts into the lower border of the thyroid lamina. Shortening (relaxation) of the vocal folds is brought about by both the thyro-arytenoid muscles and the vocalis muscle. The thyro-arytenoid arises from the posterior surface of the thyroid cartilage and inserts into the vocal process of the arytenoid cartilage. The vocalis muscle is a deep band of muscle fibers that arise from the vocal process of the arytenoid cartilage and insert at different points into the lateral surface of the vocal ligament. Thus, the muscle fibers act in much the same way as a finger on a guitar string alters the pitch of a note.

Vascular supply of the larynx

The chief arterial supply to the larynx is derived from the laryngeal branches of the superior and inferior thyroid arteries.

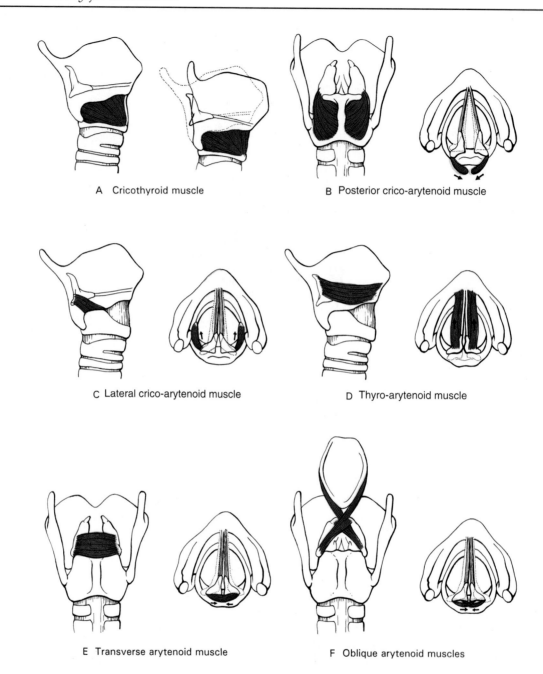

Fig. 1.30
Actions of the laryngeal muscles.

Lymphatic drainage of the larynx

The lymphatic drainage of the region of the larynx above the level of the vocal folds passes to the upper deep cervical group of lymph nodes, whereas the region below the vocal folds drains to the lower deep cervical group.

Innervation of the larynx

The innervation of the larynx is essentially vagal in origin through its superior and recurrent laryngeal branches, although there is some input from the cranial accessory through the vagus (Fig. 1.31).

The **superior laryngeal nerve** branches from the

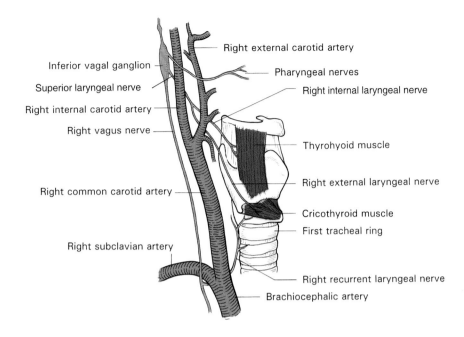

Fig. 1.31
The nerve supply of the larynx.

vagus and passes deep to both the internal and external carotid arteries before dividing into a large internal branch and a small external branch. The internal laryngeal nerve pierces the thyrohyoid membrane with the superior laryngeal artery and divides into ascending and descending branches. The ascending branch is sensory to the epiglottis and posterior part of the tongue and is responsible for supplying the taste buds in this area. The descending branch is sensory to the laryngeal mucosa down to the region of the vocal folds. In addition, it provides secretomotor fibers to the glands in the region of the saccule that are concerned with lubrication of the vocal folds. The sympathetic innervation to this region is derived from the superior cervical ganglion via fibers that follow the course of the superior laryngeal artery. The smaller external laryngeal branch from the superior laryngeal nerve carries motor fibers originating from the cranial accessory nerve. The external laryngeal nerve runs with the superior thyroid artery, lies on the inferior constrictor and then runs deep to it, piercing and supplying the muscle, before innervating the cricothyroid muscle.

The **recurrent laryngeal nerve** has a different course on each side of the body. The right recurrent laryngeal nerve leaves the vagus as it crosses the subclavian artery, loops under it and ascends to the larynx in the groove between the esophagus and the trachea. On the left-hand side, the nerve leaves the vagus as it crosses the arch of the aorta, then loops under the aorta (posterior to the ligamentum arteriosum) and ascends towards the larynx in the tracheo-esophageal groove. The right and left nerves now follow the same course and pass deep to the inferior constrictor to enter the larynx behind the cricothyroid joint, where they pierce the cricothyroid membrane. The recurrent laryngeal is the sole motor supply to all the intrinsic muscles of the larynx except the cricothyroid. Although the nerve fibers originate from the cranial accessory nerve, they are distributed via the vagus. In addition, the vagus is sensory to the laryngeal mucosa below the level of the vocal folds and secretomotor to the glands of the lower regions of the larynx. The sympathetic innervation below the level of the vocal folds is derived from the middle cervical ganglion via branches of the inferior laryngeal artery.

SOMATIC INNERVATION OF THE LARYNX

Sensory	Vagus (X) via internal laryngeal nerve to mucosa above vocal folds and recurrent laryngeal nerve → mucosa below vocal folds
Motor	Accessory (XI) distributed through vagus (X) via recurrent laryngeal nerve to all intrinsic muscles *except* cricothyroid (external laryngeal nerve to X)
Taste	Vagus (X) to epiglottis and back of tongue

26 | THE TRACHEA AND BRONCHIAL TREE

The **trachea** is a wide fibrocartilaginous tube that commences at the inferior border of the cricoid cartilage (C6) and bifurcates into the right and left principal bronchi at about the level of the sternal angle (T4/T5), with the level of the termination depending upon the phase of respiration. The trachea is, therefore, both a cervical and a thoracic structure with approximately equal lengths in each anatomical region. It can be palpated in the neck and traced from the inferior border of the cricoid cartilage to the superior border of the manubrium, where it deviates slightly to the right of the midline as it passes into the superior mediastinum.

The trachea must remain patent at all times to permit uninterrupted air flow. This is achieved by the presence of some 16–20 rings of hyaline cartilage embedded in its fibrous walls. The cartilaginous rings are deficient posteriorly and are therefore said to be 'C' shaped. This renders both flexibility and rigidity to the trachea and ensures that it is capable of withstanding fluctuations in air pressure as well as permitting the bolus of food to pass unhindered down the esophagus. As the cartilages are hyaline in nature, there is a tendency for ossification to occur with increasing age. The free posterior limits of each cartilage are connected by the trachealis muscle, which is composed of smooth (non-striated) muscle fibers.

Trachestomy may be necessary to relieve laryngeal obstruction or to permit prolonged artificial ventilation. The procedure is by no means a minor operation and, particularly in an emergency situation, it is vital to remember to remain *exactly* in the midline, as it is possible to miss the trachea entirely (Fig. 1.32). The neck should be extended and the second or third tracheal ring identified (1.5–2 cm inferior to the lower border of the cricoid cartilage). A transverse incision may be made at this level (normally the midpoint of the cricoid and the suprasternal notch) or alternatively a vertical incision made downwards from the cricoid cartilage passing between the anterior jugular veins. A hook may be placed under the lower border of the cricoid to immobilize the trachea and to pull it forward. The pretracheal fascia is split longitudinally, the isthmus of the thyroid gland is divided and the cartilages of the trachea exposed. An opening in the anterior tracheal wall is then made, avoiding the first tracheal cartilage, as damage to this structure is associated with the later development of stenosis. It should be remembered that in children the neck is relatively short, the left brachiocephalic vein may extend above the suprasternal notch, and the trachea is softer and more mobile, making it more difficult to locate. In contrast, in the elderly the tracheal rings may

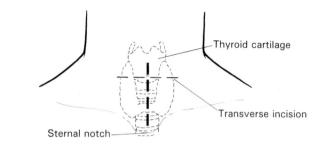

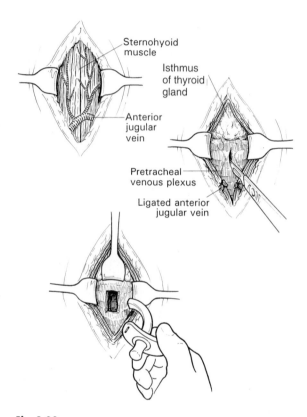

Fig. 1.32
Tracheostomy.

ossify and strong scissors may be required to open the anterior wall. Various methods of fashioning the tracheal opening have been used, mainly with the aim of minimizing the difficulty of replacing a tube which might be dislodged before a well-defined tracheotomy tract develops. If a flap or inverted U is used, care must be taken not to allow this to be pushed into the tracheal lumen when placing the tube.

Relations (Figs 1.33, 1.34 and 1.35)

Cervical

Anteriorly – skin, fascia, infrahyoid muscles, jugular arch, anterior jugular vein, isthmus of the thyroid gland covering the upper tracheal rings and if present, thyroidea ima artery,

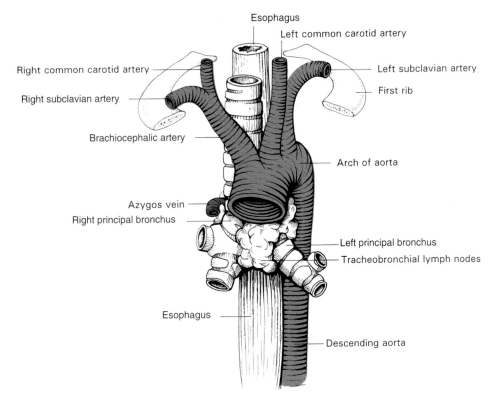

Fig. 1.33
Immediate relations of the trachea and principal bronchi.

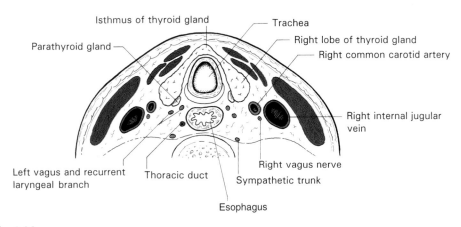

Fig. 1.34
Cross-section at the C7 vertebral level.

Posteriorly – esophagus

Laterally – recurrent laryngeal nerve in the groove between the trachea and the esophagus, the lobes of the thyroid gland down to around the sixth tracheal ring and the common carotid arteries.

Thoracic

Anteriorly – manubrium, thymus, left brachiocephalic vein, arch of the aorta, brachiocephalic and left common carotid arteries and the deep cardiac plexus

Posteriorly – esophagus

Right – right lung and pleurae, right brachiocephalic vein, superior vena cava, right vagus nerve and the azygos vein,

Left – arch of the aorta, left common carotid and left subclavian arteries.

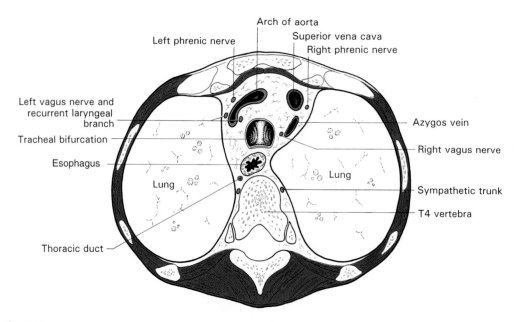

Fig. 1.35
Cross-section at the T4 vertebral level.

The trachea bifurcates into the **right** and **left principal bronchi** at the level of the fourth and fifth thoracic vertebrae (Fig. 1.36). The last tracheal cartilage is thicker and broader than the rest, with a lower border that is prolonged down and backwards in a hooked process. This forms an internal ridge known as the carina, which is visible on bronchoscopy. Each principal bronchus runs from the bifurcation of the trachea to the hilum of the lung before terminating as lobar bronchi. The right principal bronchus is shorter, wider and more vertical than the left, and as a result foreign matter is more likely to become trapped in the right bronchus. The azygos vein arches over the right principal bronchus, whilst the right pulmonary artery lies at first in front of, and then passes anterior to it. The right principal bronchus gives off its first branch (upper lobar bronchus) before it enters the hilum of the lung at the level of the fifth thoracic vertebra. In contrast, the left principal bronchus gives off no branches before entering the hilum of the left lung at the level of the sixth thoracic vertebra. It passes to the left of the arch of the aorta and crosses anterior to the esophagus, thoracic duct and descending aorta.

The right principal bronchus terminates in 3 lobar bronchi – upper, middle and lower – to supply the upper, middle and lower lobes respectively of the right lung. The left principal bronchus terminates in 2 lobar bronchi – upper and lower – which supply, respectively, the upper and lower lobes of the left lung. Variations do occur to this pattern, with the left principal bronchus occasionally terminating in 3 lobar bronchi as for the right lung.

Each lobar bronchus then terminates in **segmental bronchi** that supply each bronchopulmonary segment of the lung (Fig. 1.37 A and B). In the right lung the lobar bronchi terminate as follows:

Upper – apical, anterior and posterior segmental bronchi

Middle – lateral and medial segmental bronchi

Lower – superior, medial basal, anterior basal, lateral basal and posterior basal segmental bronchi.

The left lobar bronchi generally terminate as follows:

Upper – apical, posterior, anterior, superior lingual and inferior lingual segmental bronchi

Lower – superior, medial basal, anterior basal, lateral basal and posterior basal segmental bronchi.

The bronchial cartilages are fully formed in the extrapulmonary regions but, once intrapulmonary, the plates of cartilage become less organized until they disappear at the commencement of the bronchioles.

PLEURAE

Each lung is enveloped in a pleural sac that can best be imagined in the following way (Fig. 1.38). If your fist is the lung, imagine it being pushed into a balloon that has been partly blown up and tied. The outer surface of the balloon that is not in contact with your fist represents the outer layer of the pleural sac, the parietal pleura. The inner surface of the balloon that covers your fist represents the inner layer of the pleural sac and is the visceral pleura. The inner surface of the balloon dips down into the cracks between your fingers, as the viscera pleural dips down into the fissures between the lobes of the lung. The space

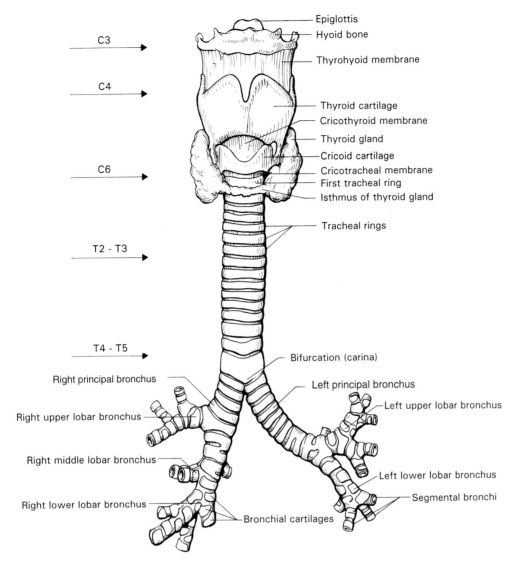

C3

C4

C6

T2 - T3

T4 - T5

Epiglottis
Hyoid bone
Thyrohyoid membrane

Thyroid cartilage
Cricothyroid membrane
Thyroid gland
Cricoid cartilage
Cricotracheal membrane
First tracheal ring
Isthmus of thyroid gland

Tracheal rings

Bifurcation (carina)

Right principal bronchus
Left principal bronchus
Left upper lobar bronchus
Right upper lobar bronchus

Right middle lobar bronchus

Left lower lobar bronchus
Segmental bronchi
Right lower lobar bronchus
Bronchial cartilages

Fig. 1.36
The trachea and bronchial tree.

between the outer and inner layers of the balloon is filled with air, but in the case of the pleural sacs this is only a potential space, as it is a vacuum where the surfaces are moistened by a thin layer of pleural fluid, which lubricates the pleural surfaces permitting friction-free movement during respiration. Where your fist has entered the balloon, the outer and inner layers become continuous, similarly, the parietal pleura is continuous with the visceral pleura at the hilum of the lung. If you now drag your fist upwards, the shape of the hilum changes and in the lung this area hangs down rather like a cuff on a jacket and is known as the pulmonary ligament. This is dead space at the hilum that permits not only descent of the hilum of the lung during descent of the diaphragm in deep inspiration, but also extension of the pulmonary veins during periods of increased vascular activity.

The parietal pleura is connected to the walls of the thorax by a loose endothoracic fascia. The parietal pleura is given different names according to the different structures to which it is related. The costal pleura covers the internal surfaces of the sternum, costal cartilages, ribs, intercostal muscles and the sides of the thoracic vertebrae. The mediastinal pleura covers the mediastinal area between the two pleural sacs. The diaphragmatic pleura covers the superior surface of the diaphragm and the cervical pleura covers the apex of the lung and passes above the midline of the clavicle into the root of the neck. This dome of pleura (cupola) is strengthened by a fibrous layer of dense fascia (suprapleural membrane) which is attached to the internal border of the first rib and the anterior border of the transverse process of the seventh cervical vertebra.

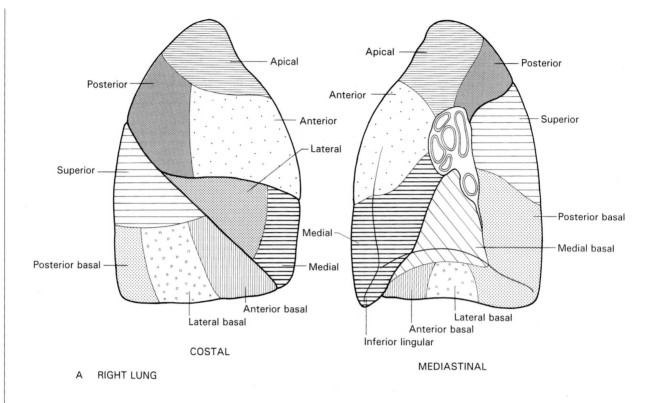

A   RIGHT LUNG

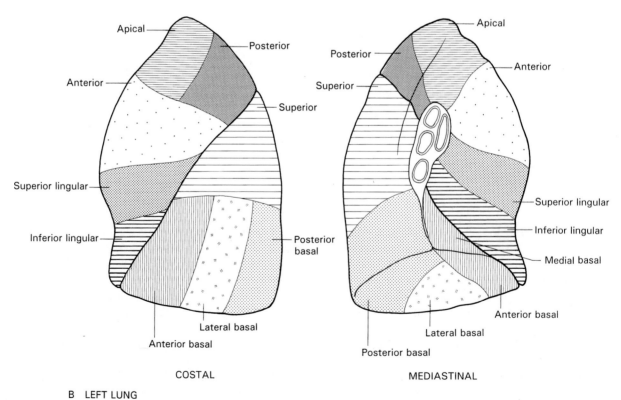

B   LEFT LUNG

Fig. 1.37
Bronchopulmonary segments of the right lung
and left lung.

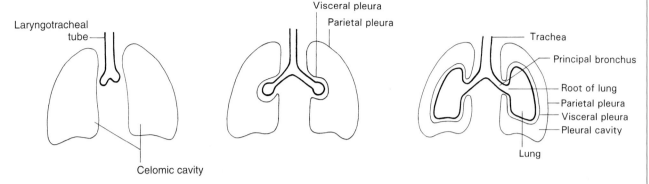

Fig. 1.38
Development of the lungs and pleural cavities.

The limits of the pleural sacs and the reflections of the parietal pleura can be mapped on the surface of the thorax (Fig. 1.39 A–D). Passing from the cupola, the anterior margins of the pleura descend obliquely behind the sternoclavicular joints to reach the midline at the level of the sternal angle. Here the two pleural sacs come in contact and may overlap slightly, each maintaining an essentially midline position down to the level of the fourth costal cartilage. The two sacs then follow a marginally different course, with the right maintaining its descent virtually in the midline before deviating laterally at the level of the xiphisternal joint. At the fourth costal cartilage, the left pleural sac deviates to the lateral border of the sternum and then descends to the seventh costal cartilage at the level of the xiphisternal joint. Both pleural sacs then follow the course of the seventh costal cartilage with the lines of reflection crossing the eighth rib at the midclavicular line, the tenth rib at the midaxillary line and passing under the neck of the twelfth rib to reach the sides of the vertebral column. From here, the lines of reflection turn upwards along the sides of the vertebral bodies to reach the cervical pleura above.

During deep inspiration, the lungs virtually fill the pleural cavities but during normal respiration parts of these cavities are unoccupied, so that areas of the parietal pleura come into direct contact. These potential spaces are the pleural recesses. The costodiaphragmatic recess is a slit-like space between the costal and diaphragmatic pleurae. A similar potential cleft exists behind the sternum, where costal and mediastinal pleurae come into contact forming the costomediastinal recess. This is clearly larger on the left than on the right due to the deviation of the anterior border of the lung at the cardiac notch.

THE LUNGS

The lungs, which are the principal organs of respiration, are enclosed within their pleural sacs and separated by the structures in the mediastinum. Their shape is largely dictated by the structures immediately surrounding them and the size of the thoracic cavity. They are conical – each has an apex, base, root or hilum, 3 surfaces and 3 borders.

The **apex** of the lung extends through the superior thoracic aperture into the root of the neck. It lies in close proximity to the cupola of the pleura and the suprapleural membrane, which is crossed by the subclavian artery leaving a groove on the mediastinal aspect of the lung.

The **base** of the lung is concave, being reciprocal in shape to the dome of the diaphragm. As the right dome of the diaphragm is higher than the left (due to the position of the liver) the diaphragmatic surface of the right lung is of a deeper concavity.

The **root** or hilum is the site where structures enter and leave the lung. It is the region where the parietal and visceral pleurae become continuous and also where the pulmonary ligament is found (Figs 1.40 and 1.41). The root is formed by the principal bronchus, pulmonary artery, pulmonary veins, bronchial arteries and veins, pulmonary plexuses of nerves and the lymphatic vessels and nodes. The superior vena cava and the right atrium lie in front of the root of the right lung and the azygos vein arches above it. The root of the left lung is ventral to the thoracic aorta and inferior to its arch. Ventral to both roots are the phrenic nerves, pericardiacophrenic vessels and the anterior pulmonary plexuses of nerves. Dorsal to the roots lie the vagus nerves and the posterior pulmonary plexuses.

There is a general correspondence on both sides concerning the entrance position of the major structures passing into the lungs. The superior pulmonary veins are ventral, the bronchi are dorsal and the pulmonary arteries lie between them. The superior–inferior relations differ on the two sides, with the upper lobar bronchus being most superior on the right side and the pulmonary artery most superior on

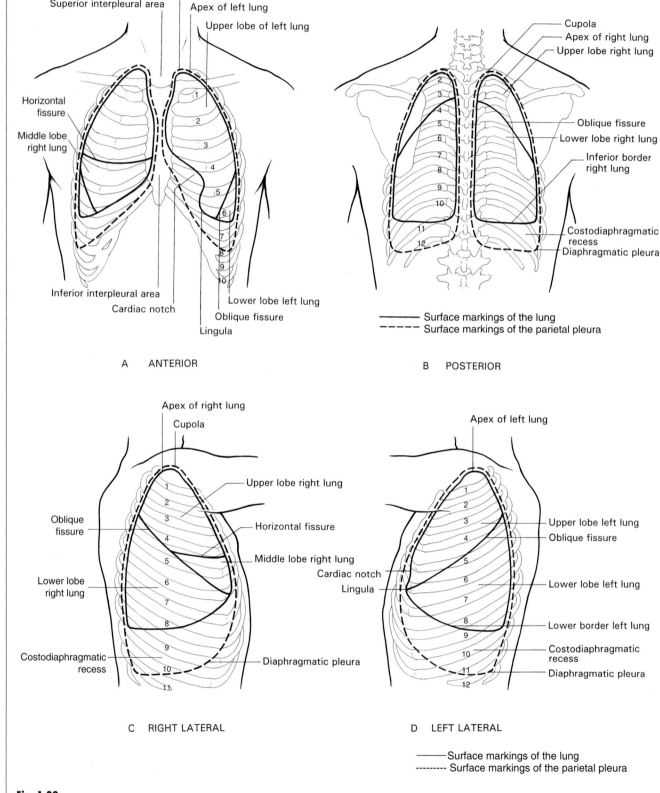

Fig. 1.39
Surface markings of the lungs and pleurae.

the left side. The veins are generally inferior and the inferior pulmonary vein is dorsal.

The right and left lungs differ in size, shape and lobular construction. Each lobe of the lung is made up of separate segments which are similar in both lungs. These bronchopulmonary segments are roughly pyramidal in shape, with their apices directed towards the hilum of the lung and their bases towards the lung surface and they are named in accordance with the

segmental bronchus that supplies them (see above). In terms of its air passage, each bronchopulmonary segment can be considered an independent structural unit and, although each segment is virtually independent in terms of its arterial supply, its venous drainage is not so clearly defined.

The right lung (Fig. 1.40) is larger and heavier than the left which has to accommodate the heart and pericardium trespassing into its space. The right lung is

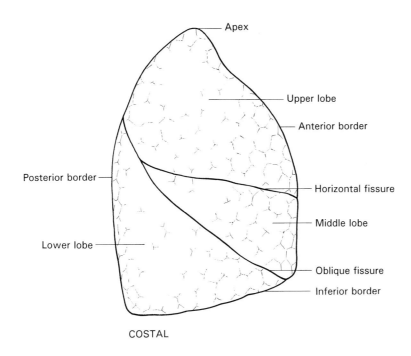

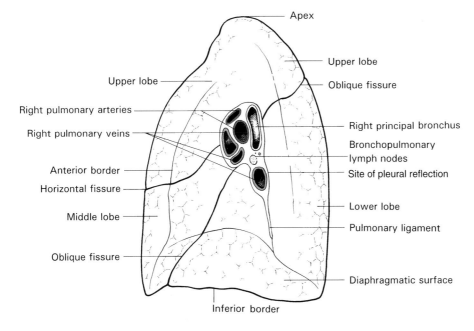

Fig. 1.40
The costal and mediastinal surfaces of the right lung.

divided into upper, middle and lower lobes which are separated by 2 fissures. The horizontal fissure separates the upper and middle lobes and the oblique fissure separates the lower from the middle and upper lobes. The left lung (Fig. 1.41) generally has 2 lobes – upper and lower – which are separated by a long and deep oblique fissure.

Each lung has 3 surfaces, costal, mediastinal and diaphragmatic, which are covered by visceral pleura that dips down into each fissure. The costal surface is large and convex and follows the contours of the lateral thoracic wall (ribs, costal cartilages and their intercostal muscles). The posterior part of this surface is related to the thoracic vertebrae and is therefore sometimes referred to as the vertebral surface. The mediastinal surface is medial and concave, reflecting the contents of the middle mediastinum (heart and pericardium). The pericardial concavity is obviously deeper on the left

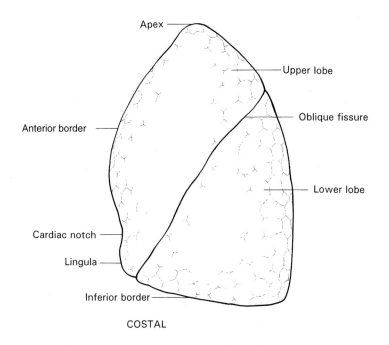

COSTAL

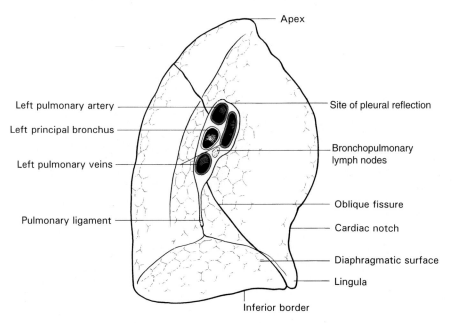

MEDIASTINAL

Fig. 1.41
The costal and mediastinal surfaces of the left lung.

lung where the heart and its major vessels leave an imprint. The mediastinal surface also contains the root of the lung around which the pleura forms the pulmonary ligament. The diaphragmatic surface is deeply concave and forms the base of the lung.

Each lung has an anterior, posterior and inferior border. The anterior border is thin and sharp and overlaps the pericardium. The left bears an indentation called the cardiac notch, which reflects displacement of the lung due to the position of the heart. A flap-like area of the lung called the lingula hangs below the cardiac notch on the left lung. The anterior border separates the costal from the mediastinal surface and more or less corresponds in position to the anterior border of the pleura. The posterior border is broad and rounded and lies in the deep paravertebral gutters lateral to the vertebral column. The inferior border circumscribes the diaphragmatic surface of the lung and separates this from the costal surface. It is thin and sharp where it projects into the costodiaphragmatic recess but is more blunt and rounded anteriorly where it separates the diaphragmatic from the mediastinal surface.

As with the pleurae, the surface markings of the lungs can be mapped on the thorax, although the surface projection is not constant due to the cycle of expansion and contraction during respiration. The apex is represented by a line drawn superiolaterally from the sternoclavicular joint to a point 2.5 cm superior to the medial third of the clavicle and inferolaterally to the junction of the middle and lateral thirds of the clavicle. The anterior borders correspond to the sternal lines of the pleural reflections except at the cardiac notch on the left, where the anterior border deviates laterally to a point approximately 2.5 cm lateral to the left edge of the sternum. It then turns inferiorly and slightly medially to the sixth left costal cartilage. The inferior borders are indicated by a line drawn from the inferior end of the line representing the anterior border that crosses the sixth rib in the midclavicular line, the eighth rib in the midaxillary line and the tenth rib approaching the vertebral column. Thus, the surface markings of the inferior border lie some 2 ribs superior to those of the pleural reflections.

The surface location of the oblique fissure is more or less the same for both right and left lungs and coincides with the medial border of the scapula when the upper limb is fully abducted at the shoulder joint. It also corresponds with a line that runs from the spinous process of the second thoracic vertebra to the sixth costochondral junction. The horizontal fissure on the right is indicated by a line that runs from the anterior border of the lung along the fourth costal cartilage until it intersects with that of the oblique fissure.

THE DIAPHRAGM

The diaphragm is the chief muscle of respiration and is a central musculofascial sheet which separates the thoracic from the abdominal cavities (Fig. 1.42). It has a central tendinous region and peripheral musculature. The muscular regions are dome-shaped, with their

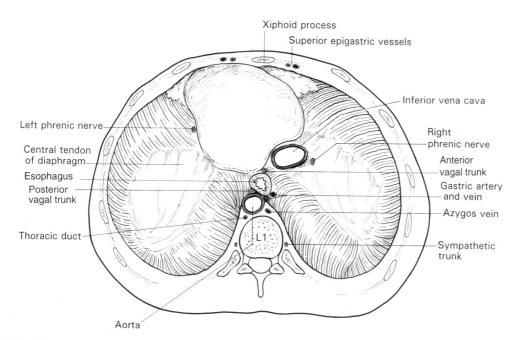

Fig. 1.42
The thoracic surface of the diaphragm.

convexity bulging into the thoracic cavity. In normal expiration the domes may reach as high as the fifth rib on the right side and the fifth intercostal space on the left. The right dome of the diaphragm is higher due to the mass of the liver. The central tendon is described as trefoil in shape and associated musculature radiates from the sternum, ribs, costal cartilages and sides of the upper lumbar vertebrae towards the central tendon. The diaphragm has 4 major openings that permit the passage of structures to and from the thoracic and abdominal cavities:

1. *Aortic hiatus* – found at the level of the twelfth thoracic vertebra through which passes the aorta, the thoracic duct and sometimes the azygos vein
2. *Esophageal hiatus* – located at the level of the tenth thoracic vertebra through which passes the esophagus, left gastric artery and vein and the anterior and posterior trunks of the vagus nerve
3. *Caval hiatus* – located in the central tendinous region at the level of the eighth thoracic vertebra and transmits the inferior vena cava with branches of the right phrenic nerve and lymphatic vessels
4. *Sternocostal hiatus* – this is a small interval between adjacent sternal and costal origins of the diaphragmatic muscular origins and transmits lymphatic vessels from the liver to the anterior phrenic nodes as well as the superior epigastric artery.

MECHANISM OF RESPIRATION

Respiration requires a change in thoracic pressure, which is mediated by alterations in thoracic dimensions. These changes in dimensions occur:

1. In the superior–inferior direction, by active descent of the diaphragm and elevation of the first rib manubrium complex. On inspiration the domes of the diaphragm descend and, in addition, the rigid bar formed by the first rib, its costal cartilage and the manubrium are elevated by the action of the scalene muscles
2. Anteroposteriorly, by movements of the sternum at the manubriosternal joint brought about by the pincer-like action of the lower ribs
3. Laterally, by the excursions of the ribs acting in a 'bucket handle'-like motion brought about by the obliquity of the rib shaft.

During quiet inspiration, the diaphragm accounts for most of the muscular activity associated with respiration, although the scalene muscles do play a minor role. In forced inspiration, the diaphragm undergoes maximal contraction along with action in the spinal erectors and muscles connecting the upper limb to the trunk, e.g. the pectorals. Quiet expiration occurs primarily by elastic recoil of the lungs and thoracic wall with a slow relaxation of the inspiratory muscles. Forced expiration, such as sneezing and coughing, is accompanied by strong contraction of the abdominal and the latissimus dorsi muscles.

Vascular supply of the lower respiratory tract

The cervical region of the trachea derives its arterial supply from branches of the inferior thyroid artery, whilst the lower regions and bronchial tree are supplied by the bronchial arteries which arise from the descending thoracic aorta and the upper intercostal arteries. The parietal pleura derives its arterial supply from body wall sources, e.g. the intercostal, internal thoracic and musculophrenic arteries. The visceral pleura and lungs are supplied by the bronchial arteries. The diaphragm is supplied by branches from the musculophrenic and superior epigastric arteries and via phrenic branches from the thoracic aorta.

Lymphatic drainage of the lower respiratory tract

The lymph vessels from the trachea and bronchial tree pass either to the pretracheal or paratracheal group of nodes. The lymph vessels of the parietal pleura pass to the intercostal, parasternal, posterior mediastinal and diaphragmatic groups of nodes. The vessels draining lymph from the visceral pleura and lungs pass to the bronchopulmonary group of nodes. The lymphatic vessels of the diaphragm drain into 2 plexuses – one on the thoracic surface and one on the abdominal surface. The former pass to the diaphragmatic nodes and the latter to the aortic group of nodes.

INNERVATION OF THE LOWER RESPIRATORY TRACT AND DIAPHRAGM

Tracheobronchial tree

Sensory	Vagus (X) and recurrent laryngeal branches
Motor	Sympathetic trunks – bronchodilation
	Vagus (X) – bronchoconstriction

Pleurae

Parietal sensory	Phrenic and intercostal nerves
Visceral sensory	Autonomic pp. (156)

Lungs

Autonomic (pp. 156)

Diaphragm

Sensory	Lower 6 or 7 intercostal nerves
Motor	Phrenic nerve (C3-C5)

2

The cardiovascular system

The cardiovascular system comprises the heart and blood vessels, which are separated into 2 distinct components – pulmonary and systemic (Fig. 2.1). The **pulmonary** system incorporates all structures involved in transferring deoxygenated blood from the heart to the lungs and back again. Deoxygenated blood passes into the right atrium, then to the right ventricle via the tricuspid valve, and is pumped out via the pulmonary trunk and pulmonary arteries to the lungs (Fig. 2.2). Following oxygenation, blood returns to the left atrium via the pulmonary veins. The **systemic** system incorporates all structures involved in conveying oxygenated blood from the heart to the tissues of the body. Oxygenated blood enters the left atrium, passes through the mitral valve into the left ventricle, and is pumped into the aorta and thence to all tissues of the body.

Blood vessels are named in accordance with the direction of the blood flow and not with the degree of oxygenation. Thus, all arteries carry blood *away* from the heart (e.g. pulmonary arteries, aorta etc.) and all veins convey blood *towards* the heart (e.g. pulmonary veins, subclavian veins etc).

THE HEART

The heart sits in the middle mediastinum of the thorax (Figs. 2.3, 2.X1 and 2.X2), posterior to the sternum and costal cartilages and anterior to thoracic vertebrae 5–8. It is enclosed in a fibroserous sac, the pericardium, which covers both the heart and the roots of the great vessels. The **fibrous pericardium** is a tough outer sac whose apex is pierced by the aorta, pulmonary trunk and superior vena cava. The base of the fibrous pericardium rests on, and fuses with, the central tendon of the diaphragm, whilst its apex extends up to the level of the sternal angle around the ascending aorta. Anteriorly it is attached to the dorsum of the sternum by sternopericardial ligaments.

The **serous pericardium** has 2 components: the parietal pericardium and the visceral pericardium. The **parietal** layer of the serous pericardium lines the inner surface of the fibrous layer and becomes continuous with the **visceral pericardium** (which is in direct contact with the heart surface) around the bases of the great vessels. A potential space exists between the parietal and visceral layer, and this is the pericardial cavity which contains a thin film of viscous fluid. During the foldings of the embryonic heart, sinuses are formed in the pericardium. The **transverse pericardial sinus** is located posterior to the ascending aorta and pulmonary trunk and anterior to the great veins, whilst the **oblique sinus** occurs at the base of the heart, posterior to the left atrium.

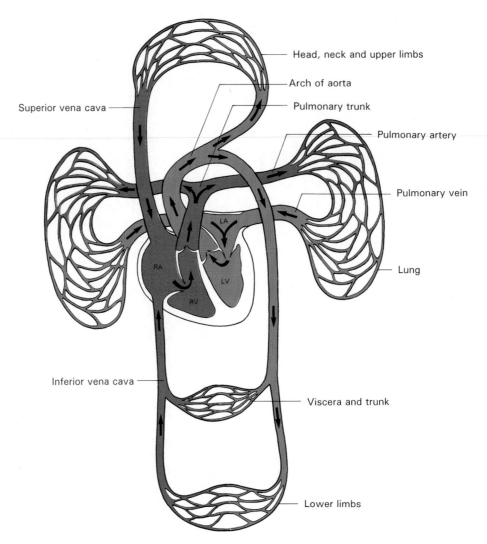

Fig. 2.1
The principles of cardiovascular flow.

The arterial supply to the fibrous and parietal pericardium arises from the pericardiacophrenic and musculophrenic branches of the internal thoracic artery, along with branches from the bronchial, esophageal and superior phrenic arteries. The visceral pericardium receives its arterial supply from the coronary arteries. The veins from the pericardium drain into the azygos system and the internal thoracic vein. The innervation is via the vagus, phrenic and sympathetic trunks.

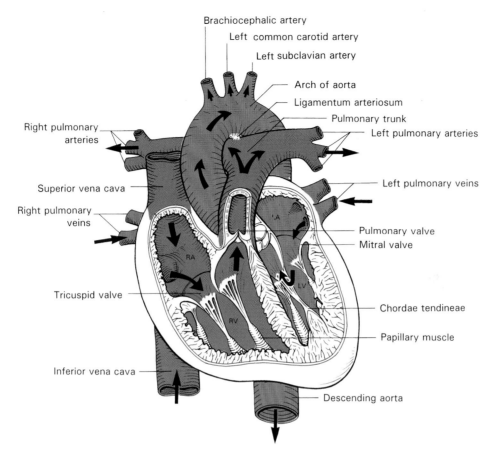

Fig. 2.2
Direction of blood flow in the heart and great vessels.

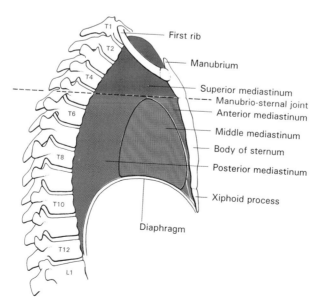

Fig. 2.3
The divisions of the mediastinum.

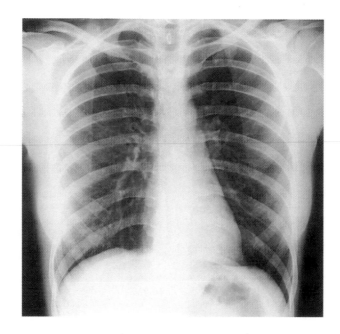

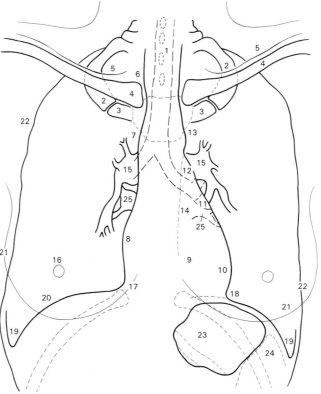

Fig. 2.X1

Normal postero-anterior chest radiograph with line diagram.

1 Air in trachea	10 Left ventricle	18 Left cardiophrenic angea
2 First rib	11 Left auricle (auricular	19 Lateral costophrenic aorta
3 First costal cartilage	appendage of left atrium)	20 Right cupola of diaphram
4 Clavicles	12 Pulmonary trunk (conus)	21 Breast shadow
5 Skin line over clavicles	13 Aortic knuckle or knob	22 Lateral border of thoracic
6 Right brachiocephalic vein	14 Lateral border of descending	cage
(innominate vein)	thoracic aorta	23 Fundal air bubble
7 Superior vena cava	15 Pulmonary artery	24 Spleen
8 Right atrium	16 Right nipple	25 Pulmonary veins
9 Right ventricle	17 Inferior vena cava	

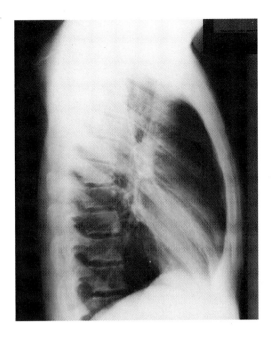

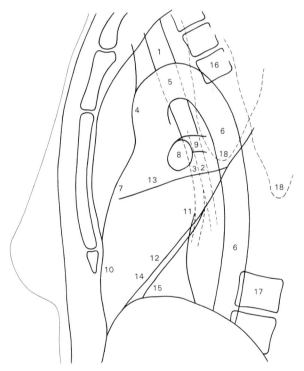

Fig. 2.X2
Normal lateral chest radiograph with line diagram.

1 Trachea
2 Left main bronchus
3 Right main bronchus
4 Ascending thoracic aorta
5 Aortic arch
6 Descending thoracic aorta
7 Pulmonary outflow tract

8 Right main pulmonary artery
9 Left main pulmonary artery
10 Site of right ventricle
11 Site of left atrium
12 Site of left ventricle

13 Horizontal fissure
14 Right oblique fissure
15 Left oblique fissure
16 Vertebral body of T4
17 Vertebral body of T11
18 Inferior angle of scapula

Surface anatomy

The heart possesses a base, an apex, anterior and inferior surfaces and right and left borders (Figs 2.4 and 2.5). The **base** of the heart is quadrilateral in shape and is located posteriorly, being formed mainly by the left atrium. It lies opposite thoracic vertebrae 6–9 and faces superiorly, posteriorly and to the right. The **apex** of the heart is primarily formed from the left ventricle and is located posterior to the left fifth intercostal space some 7–9 cm from the midline. The **anterior** surface, also known as the sternocostal surface, lies posterior to the sternum and the costal cartilages and is primarily formed from the right ventricle. The **inferior** surface, also known as the diaphragmatic surface, rests on the central tendon of the thoracic diaphragm and is made up of both the right and left ventricles. The **left border** of the heart occupies the cardiac notch of the left lung and is primarily formed from the left ventricle, whereas the **right border** is almost entirely right atrial in origin.

The surface markings of the borders of the heart are (Fig. 2.6):

Superior
Right 3rd costal cartilage, 2 cm from midline → left 2nd costal cartilage, 3 cm from midline.

Right
Right 3rd costal cartilage, 2 cm from midline → right 6th costal cartilage, 2 cm from midline.

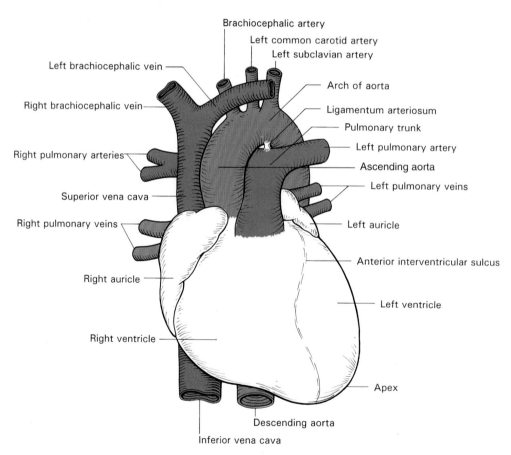

Fig. 2.4
The sternocostal surface of the heart.

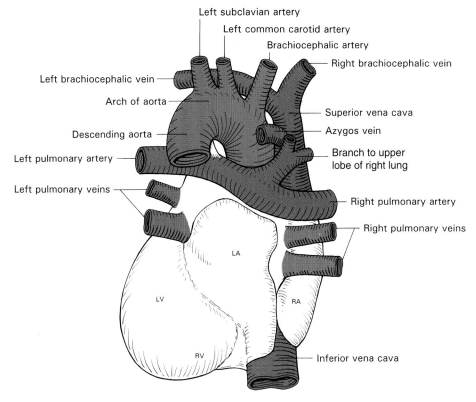

Fig. 2.5
The base of the heart.

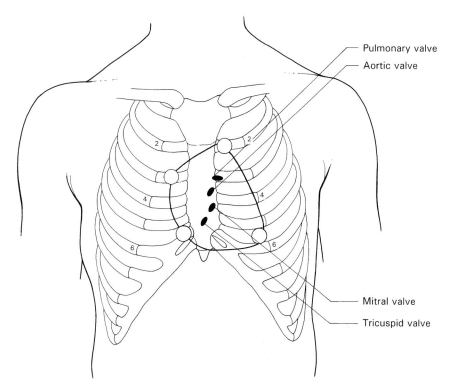

Fig. 2.6
Surface markings of the borders and valves of the heart.

Inferior
Right 6th costal cartilage, 2 cm from midline → left 5th intercostal space, 7 cm from midline.

Left
Left 5th intercostal space, 7 cm from midline → left 2nd costal cartilage, 2 cm from midline.

Chambers of the heart (Figs 2.7–2.10)

The **right atrium** receives deoxygenated venous blood from all body tissues via the superior and inferior venae cavae and from the heart tissue itself via the coronary sinus and the small independent veins that open directly into its cavity. The posterior aspect of the right atrium is derived from the embryological right horn of the sinus venosus and the primitive atrium (see below). These two distinct derivative components can be distinguished by the presence of a muscular ridge (crista terminalis) that extends between the orifices for the superior and inferior venae cavae. Muscular ridges (musculi pectinati) extend forward from the crista and pass across the lateral and anterior walls of the atrium towards the tricuspid orifice and these are important in atrial systole. The sinu-atrial node or 'pacemaker' of the

heart (see page 45) is situated in the upper part of the crista, whilst the atrioventricular node lies at the junction between the interatrial septum and the base of the tricuspid valve. The interatrial wall has an oval depression (fossa ovalis) which represents the remnants of the foramen ovale of the fetal heart.

The **right ventricle** extends from the tricuspid opening to the conus arteriosus (infundibulum) and then to the pulmonary orifice. The blood flow through the ventricle is channelled via an inflow and an outflow system which are separated by the supraventricular crest. The area of the ventricle associated with inflow has rough walls made up of bundles of muscle fibers (trabeculae carneae) which are covered by endocardium and project into the ventricular cavity. Several of these trabeculae are specialized into papillary muscles whose bases are continuous with the ventricular musculature but whose apices project into the cavity and are attached to the cusps of the atrioventricular valve by the chordae tendineae. The region of the ventricle associated with blood outflow (infundibulum) is smooth-walled and represents a persistent part of the embryological bulbus cordis (see below).

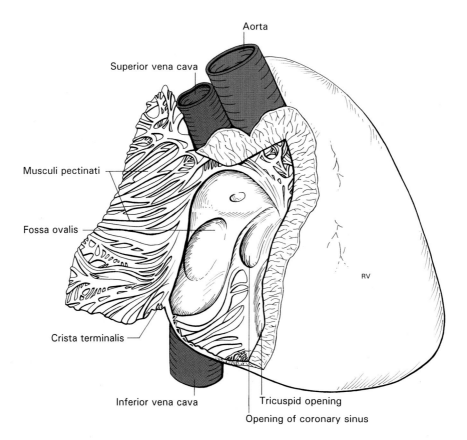

Aorta

Superior vena cava

Musculi pectinati

Fossa ovalis

Crista terminalis

Inferior vena cava

RV

Tricuspid opening

Opening of coronary sinus

Fig. 2.7
The right atrium.

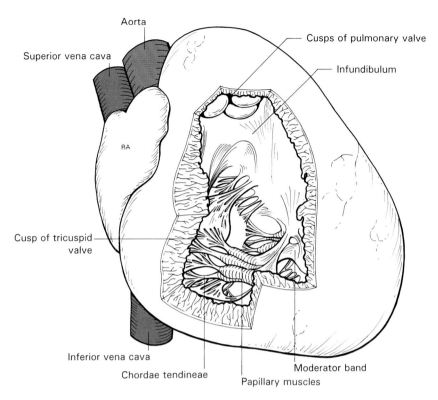

Aorta

Superior vena cava

Cusps of pulmonary valve

Infundibulum

RA

Cusp of tricuspid valve

Inferior vena cava

Chordae tendineae

Papillary muscles

Moderator band

Fig. 2.8
The right ventricle.

The **left atrium** is smaller than the right atrium but possesses thicker walls. The 4 pulmonary veins open into the upper part of its posterior surface. The musculi pectinati are fewer and smaller than those found in the right atrium, and they are confined to the region of the auricle.

The **left ventricle** also has both an inflow and an outflow pathway for blood but they pass in close contact and are not clearly separated. The muscular walls are considerably thicker than those of the right ventricle and the trabeculation is more intense. The trabeculae carneae are more robust and there are only 2 papillary muscles.

The orifice of the **tricuspid valve** is circular in outline and strengthened by an underlying ring of collagenous tissue that forms the skeleton of the heart. The 3 cusps of the valve (anterior, posterior and septal) arise from the base of the orifice and the annular ring, and pass into the ventricular cavity as a flap of tissue

covered by endocardium. The undersurface of the cusps are attached to 3 papillary muscles by the chordae tendineae.

The **pulmonary valve** is situated at the exit of the venous outflow from the right ventricle and at the junction with the pulmonary trunk. It possesses 3 cusps which are semilunar in shape and attached to the fibrous thickening of the walls of the pulmonary trunk.

The orifice of the **mitral (bicuspid) valve** is smaller than that of the tricuspid valve but it is also circular in outline. As its name implies, there are only 2 valve cusps, which attach to both the anterior and posterior papillary muscles of the left ventricle.

The **aortic valve** is situated at the base of the aorta and consists of 3 semilunar cusps whose bases attach to the fibrous skeleton of the heart. Three dilations occur behind the valves and these are the aortic sinuses, which give rise to the coronary arteries.

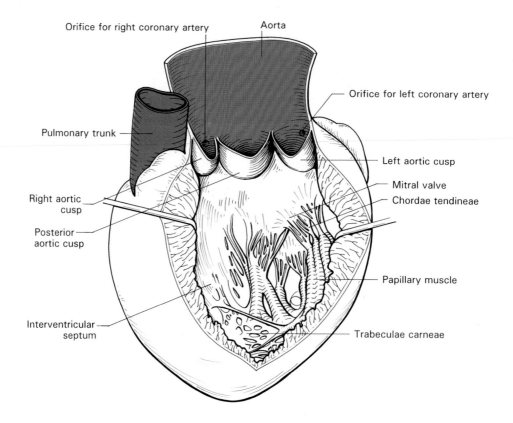

Fig. 2.9
The left ventricle.

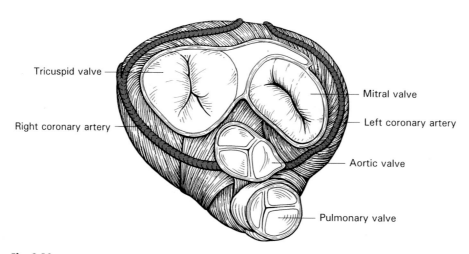

Fig. 2.10
The valves of the heart viewed from above (atria have been removed).

Electrical conduction

The electrical stimulation of the heart commences in the sinu-atrial (SA) node which is located in the superior wall of the right atrium near the entry of the superior vena cava (Fig. 2.11). This node makes contact with atrial muscle cells which causes them to depolarize, initiating a wave of electrical activity which spreads through both atria. This causes the atria to contract and propel blood into the ventricles. From the SA node, electrical activity reaches the atrioventricular (AV) node at the base of the septal wall of the right atrium adjacent to the tricuspid valve. The conducting system of the heart is not structurally continuous and electrical activity passes from the SA node to the AV node through the heart muscle fibers themselves. There is, therefore, a slight delay in electrical activity, so that the atria and ventricles do not contract in unison. From the AV node, the electrical impulse passes down the AV bundle (bundle of His) in the interventricular septum. At the base, it divides into 2 branches which pass to each of the two ventricles. At the apex of the ventricles they divide into numerous Purkinje fibres which pass directly into the muscular walls of the ventricles and so initiate contraction.

PULMONARY VESSELS

The **pulmonary trunk** conveys deoxygenated blood from the right ventricle of the heart to the alveolar tissue of the lungs. From the right ventricle, it passes upwards and backwards and is initially located in front of the ascending aorta before passing to its left (Fig. 2.4). It divides in the concavity of the aortic arch (at the level of the fifth thoracic vertebra) into the right and left pulmonary arteries. The **right pulmonary artery** is longer and larger than its left counterpart and runs horizontally to the right, passing behind the ascending aorta and in front of the esophagus. At the hilum of the right lung it divides into 2 branches. The **left pulmonary artery** passes horizontally to the left, crossing in front of the descending aorta. At the root of the left lung it too divides into 2 branches. The superior surface of the left pulmonary artery is connected to the lower border of the aortic arch above by the ligamentum arteriosum, which is the remnant of the fetal ductus arteriosus (see below).

The **pulmonary veins** convey oxygenated blood from the alveolar tissue of the lungs to the left atrium of the heart. There are generally 4 pulmonary veins (2 from each lung) and they perforate the fibrous

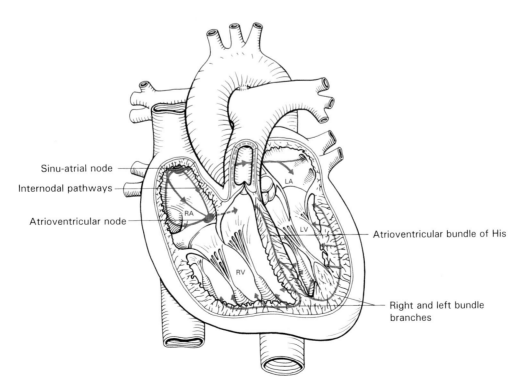

Fig. 2.11
The conducting system of the heart.

pericardium before opening independently into the left atrium (Fig. 2.5). The **right pulmonary veins** pass behind the superior vena cava to gain access to the heart, whilst the **left pulmonary veins** pass in front of the descending aorta.

SYSTEMIC VESSELS

Aorta

The aorta commences at the aortic valves and terminates opposite the fourth lumbar vertebra, where it bifurcates into the common iliac arteries (Fig. 2.12). Topographically it is separated into 4 parts – ascending, arch, descending thoracic and abdominal.

Ascending aorta

This commences at the aortic valves at the exit site from the left ventricle (Fig. 2.4). This is a short section of only some 5 cm and it is directed upwards and slightly to the right. It is continuous superiorly with the arch of the aorta, behind the manubrium and opposite the right second costal cartilage. At the base of the ascending aorta, immediately superior to the cusps of the valve, is a smooth dilation which forms the aortic sinuses. The only branches from this part of the aorta arise from the right and left coronary sinuses and these are the right and left coronary arteries respectively (Fig. 2.13).

The sulci on the external surface of the heart reflect the internal chamber organization. On the external surface the atria are separated from the ventricles by an **atrioventricular (coronary) sulcus**. Within this groove lie the main trunks of the coronary arteries. The ventricles are separated by anterior and posterior (inferior) interventricular sulci which extend from the coronary sulcus to the apical incisure of the ventricles. The **anterior interventricular sulcus** carries the anterior interventricular artery and the great cardiac vein, whilst the **posterior interventricular sulcus** carries the posterior interventricular descending artery and the middle cardiac vein.

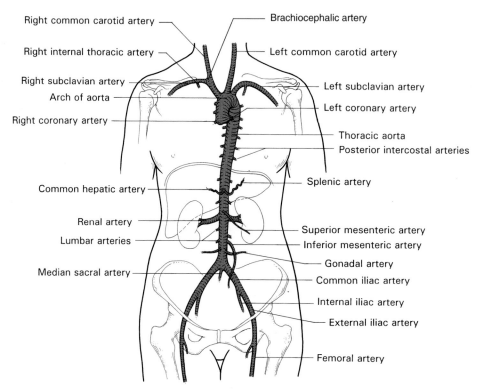

Fig. 2.12
The aorta and its principal branches.

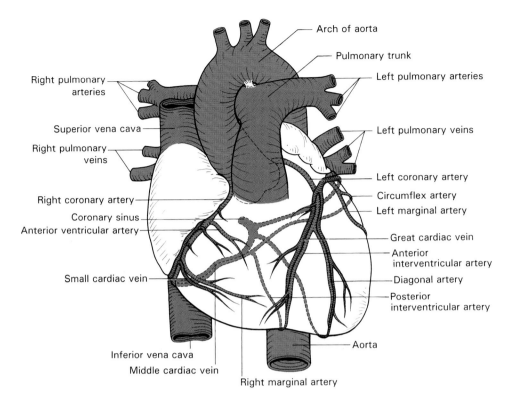

Fig. 2.13
The coronary circulation.

BRANCHES OF THE ASCENDING AORTA

	Named branch	Area of arterial supply
1. **Right coronary artery**	(1) Conus	Pulmonary conus and right ventricle
	(2) Anterior atrial branches	Right atrium
	(3) Anterior ventricular branches	Right ventricle
	(4) Marginal	Right ventricle
	(5) Posterior ventricular branches	Right ventricle
	(6) Posterior interventricular	Right and left ventricles
	(7) Artery of sinu-atrial node	Right atrium and sinu-atrial node
	(8) Septal branches	Interventricular septum
	(9) Posterior septal	Atrioventricular node
2. **Left coronary artery**	(1) Anterior interventricular	Right and left ventricles, septum
	(2) Diagonal	Left ventricle
	(3) Circumflex	Left atrium and ventricle
	(4) Marginal	Left ventricle

Arch of the aorta

The arch of the aorta is the continuation of the ascending part and it passes upwards, backwards and to the left. It is located posterior to the manubrium and it passes anterior to the trachea and over the root of the left lung before descending to the level of the fourth thoracic vertebra somewhat left of the midline. Three major branches arise from the superior border of the arch (Fig. 2.12):

1. brachiocephalic
2. left common carotid
3. left subclavian.

A small fourth branch, the thyroidea ima artery, may also arise from the arch and it passes to the isthmus of the thyroid gland. On the left-hand side, the arch is crossed by the left phrenic nerve and the left vagus which gives off the recurrent laryngeal nerve that hooks under the arch before ascending to the larynx.

BRANCHES OF THE ARCH OF THE AORTA

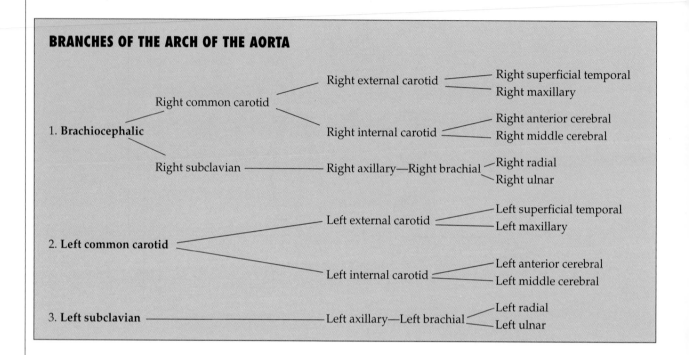

Descending thoracic aorta

This commences opposite the fourth thoracic vertebra and terminates at the aortic opening in the diaphragm opposite the last thoracic vertebra. From this portion of the aorta, paired posterior intercostal arteries pass to the body wall, paired bronchial arteries supply respiratory tissue, and midline esophageal branches supply the esophagus.

BRANCHES OF THE DESCENDING THORACIC AORTA

	Named branch	Area of arterial supply
1. **Visceral**	(1) Pericardial	Pericardium
	(2) Bronchial	Bronchial and lung tissue
	(3) Esophageal	Esophagus
	(4) Mediastinal	Posterior mediastinum
	(5) Phrenic	Posterior of diaphragm
2. **Somatic**	Posterior intercostals:	
	Dorsal	Vertebrae, spinal cord, meninges, skin and muscle of the back
	Muscular	Intercostals, pectorals, serratus anterior
	Lateral cutaneous	Skin at side of thorax
	Mammary	Breast

Abdominal aorta

This commences at the aortic opening in the diaphragm opposite the last thoracic vertebra and terminates at the bifurcation into the common iliac arteries at the level of the fourth lumbar vertebra. The abdominal aorta is virtually in the midline superiorly but deviates slightly to the left as it descends to its termination. It gives off three types of branches:

1. paired lumbar arteries to supply the body wall

2. paired visceral (non-gut) arteries–inferior phrenic, suprarenal, renal and gonadal
3. unpaired midline arteries that supply the derivatives of:
   – the embryonic foregut (celiac trunk, Fig. 2.14)
   – the embryonic midgut (superior mesenteric artery, Fig. 2.15)
   – the embryonic hindgut (inferior mesenteric artery, Fig. 2.16).

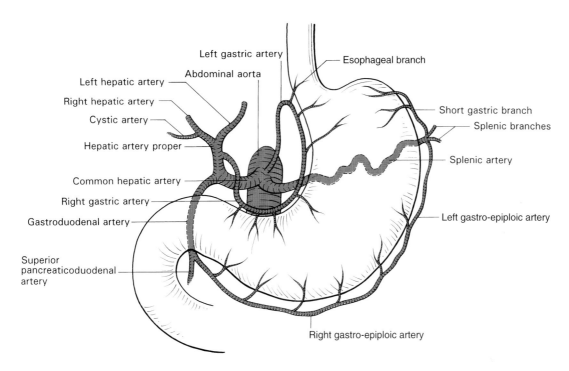

Fig. 2.14
The distribution of the celiac trunk.

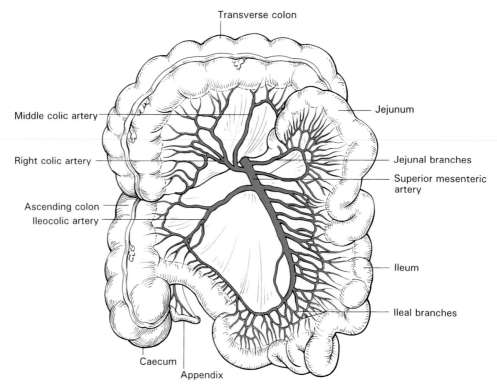

Fig. 2.15
The distribution of the superior mesenteric artery.

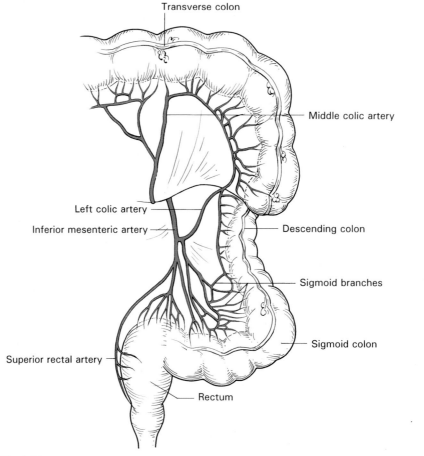

Fig. 2.16
The distribution of the inferior mesenteric artery.

BRANCHES OF THE ABDOMINAL AORTA

	Named branch	Area of arterial supply
1. **Ventral (visceral)**	(1) Celiac	Derivatives of embryonic foregut
	(2) Superior mesenteric	Derivatives of embryonic midgut
	(3) Inferior mesenteric	Derivatives of embryonic hindgut
2. **Lateral (visceral)**	(1) Inferior phrenic	Diaphragm, suprarenal gland
	(2) Middle suprarenal	Suprarenal gland
	(3) Renal	Kidney, suprarenal gland
	(4) Gonadal	Testes/ovaries, kidney, ureter
3. **Dorsal (somatic)**	(1) Lumbar	Muscles and skin of the back, vertebrae, spinal cord, meninges
	(2) Median sacral	Posterior of rectum
4. **Terminal (right and left common iliacs)**	Internal iliac	Lower GI tract, external genitalia, pelvic viscera

External iliac—Femoral—Popliteal ⟨ Anterior tibial—Dorsalis pedis
posterior tibial—Medial plantar
⟍Lateral plantar

BRANCHES OF THE CELIAC TRUNK

	Named branch	Area of arterial supply
1. **Left gastric**		Esophagus, stomach
2. **Common hepatic**	(1) Right gastric	Stomach
	(2) Gastroduodenal	Stomach, duodenum, pancreas, bile duct
	(3) Right hepatic	Liver, gall bladder
	(4) Left hepatic	Liver
3. **Splenic**	(1) Pancreatic branches	Pancreas
	(2) Short gastric	Stomach
	(3) Posterior gastric	Stomach
	(4) Left gastroepiploic	Stomach
	(5) Splenic branches	Spleen

BRANCHES OF THE SUPERIOR MESENTERIC ARTERY

1. **Inferior pancreaticoduodenal**	Pancreas, duodenum
2. **Jejunal and Ileal**	Small intestines
3. **Ileocolic**	Ascending colon, caecum, appendix, lower ileum
4. **Right colic**	Ascending colon
5. **Middle colic**	Transverse colon

54

BRANCHES OF THE INFERIOR MESENTERIC ARTERY

		Area of arterial supply
1.	**Left colic**	Transverse and descending colon
2.	**Sigmoid branches**	Sigmoid colon
3.	**Superior rectal**	Rectum

The great arteries of the neck
(Fig. 2.17)

The **brachiocephalic artery** is the first and largest of the great arteries to arise from the arch of the aorta. It passes upwards posteriorly and to the right from the midline of the arch. Behind the right sternoclavicular joint it bifurcates into the right common carotid and right subclavian arteries. There are usually no branches from the brachiocephalic artery, although in rare circumstances it may give rise to the thyroidea ima branch.

The **right common carotid artery** arises from the brachiocephalic artery posterior to the right sternoclavicular joint. It then ascends within the carotid sheath to the level of the superior border of the thyroid cartilage, where it terminates by dividing into the right internal and external carotid arteries.

The **right subclavian artery** runs from behind the right sternoclavicular joint to the lateral border of the first rib, where it becomes the axillary artery. It arches over the cervical pleura and apex of the right lung to occupy a groove on the superior surface of the first rib. Throughout its relatively short course it gives rise to 5 branches – vertebral, internal thoracic, thyrocervical, costocervical and dorsal scapular.

The **left common carotid artery** is the second branch of the arch. It ascends to the thoracic inlet passing posteriorly and slightly to the left to adopt a position posterior to the left sternoclavicular joint. The left common carotid does not usually give rise to any branches.

The **left subclavian artery** is the third and most posterior branch from the arch. It ascends behind the left common carotid to the thoracic inlet, where it arches over the cervical pleura to occupy a groove on the superior surface of the first rib. At the lateral border of this rib it becomes known as the axillary artery.

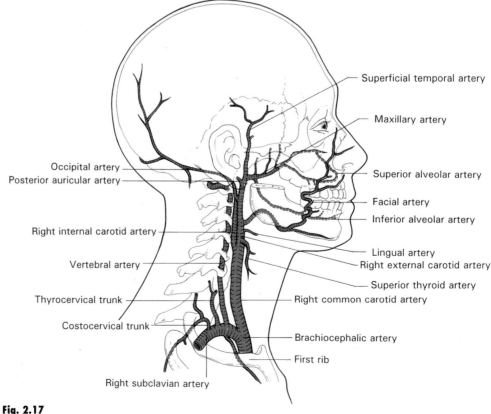

Fig. 2.17
The major arteries of the head and neck.

BRANCHES OF THE SUBCLAVIAN ARTERY

	Named branch	Area of arterial supply
1. Vertebral	(1) Spinal and muscular branches	Deep muscles of neck, spinal cord vertebrae
	(2) Meningeal branches	Dura and occipital bone
	(3) Anterior and posterior spinal	Spinal cord, meninges
	(4) Posterior inferior cerebellar	Cerebellum, medulla oblongata
2. Internal thoracic	(1) Anterior intercostal	Anterior aspect of intercostal space
	(2) Branches to	Pericardium, diaphragm, parietal pleura, sternum, thymus
3. Thyrocervical	(1) Inferior thyroid	Pharynx, larynx, trachea, esophagus, thyroid gland
	(2) Suprascapular	Muscles of back, shoulder joint, clavicle, scapula, skin of chest
	(3) Superficial cervical	Structures of posterior triangle
4. Costocervical	(1) Superior intercostal	Intercostal spaces 1 and 2
	(2) Deep cervical	Deep muscles of neck, vertebral column
5. Dorsal scapular		Muscles of back around scapula

The carotid arteries (Fig. 2.17)

Each **common carotid artery** extends upwards from behind the sternoclavicular joint to the superior border of the lamina of the thyroid cartilage. At this level, which corresponds to the fourth cervical vertebra, the common carotid bifurcates into the external and internal carotid arteries. The **external carotid artery** carries the principal blood supply to the head and neck and extends upwards from the superior border of the thyroid cartilage to a point midway between the angle of the mandible and the mastoid process. Within the parotid gland, it bifurcates into its two terminal branches: the maxillary and superficial temporal arteries. The **maxillary artery** is the larger of the two terminal branches and is the principal arterial supply to the upper and lower jaws. The **superficial temporal artery** arises deep to the neck of the mandible and is the smaller of the two terminal branches. It crosses the zygomatic arch in company with the auriculotemporal nerve and forms an extensive anastomosis in the scalp.

BRANCHES OF THE EXTERNAL CAROTID ARTERY

		Area of arterial supply
1. **Superior thyroid**		Thyroid gland, midline structures of neck, larynx
2. **Ascending pharyngeal**		Pharynx, tonsil, auditory tube, tympanic cavity, dura
3. **Lingual**		Tongue, floor of mouth, tonsil, soft palate epiglottis, sublingual gland
4. **Facial**	(1) Cervical branches	Submandibular gland, tonsil, root of tongue muscles and skin of chin and lower lip
	(2) Facial branches	Lower lip, upper lip, nasal septum, nasal ala

BRANCHES OF THE EXTERNAL CAROTID ARTERY (Contd.)

		Area of arterial supply
5. Occipital		Mastoid air cells, dura, tympanic cavity and membrane, semicircular canals, auricle, muscles and skin at back of neck and posterior scalp
6. Posterior auricular		Auricular muscles, auricle, scalp above ear
7. Superficial temporal		Parotid gland, temporomandibular joint, muscles and skin of scalp
8. Maxillary	(1) Mandibular part	External auditory meatus, tympanic membrane, temporomandibular joint, dura, pterygoid muscles, mandible, dentition
	(2) Pterygoid part	Muscles of facial expression and mastication
	(3) Pterygopalatine part	Maxilla, dentition, maxillary sinus, orbital structures, soft palate tonsil, pharynx, auditory tube, tympanic cavity, air sinuses, nasal septum

The **internal carotid artery** is the principal arterial supply to the intracranial cavity and lies lateral to the external carotid near the carotid bifurcation. It passes upwards through the cervical region without giving off any branches and enters the skull through the carotid canal before finally terminating in the interpeduncular fossa 'as' the anterior and middle cerebral arteries (see Chapter 3).

BRANCHES OF THE INTERNAL CAROTID ARTERY

	Named branch	Area of arterial supply
1. **Cervical part**	No branches	
2. **Petrous part**	(1) Caroticotympanic	Tympanic cavity
	(2) Pterygoid	Contents of pterygoid canal
3. **Cavernous part**	(1) Cavernous	Contents of cavernous sinus
	(2) Hypophyseal	Pituitary gland
	(3) Meningeal	Dura
4. **Cerebral part**	(1) Ophthalmic	Eyelids, dura, nasal cavity, retina, lacrimal gland, contents of orbit, skin and muscles of forehead, frontal and ethmoidal air sinuses
	(2) Anterior cerebral	Brain tissue
	(3) Middle cerebral	Brain tissue
	(4) Posterior communicating	Brain tissue
	(5) Anterior choroidal	Choroid plexus of lateral ventricles

The arteries of the upper limb

(Fig. 2.18)

The **axillary artery** is the continuation of the subclavian artery and extends from the lateral border of the first rib to the lower border of the teres major muscle. It is enclosed in the axillary sheath with the axillary vein and the brachial plexus. The vein lies medial to the artery, which is surrounded on appropriate sides by the medial, lateral and posterior cords of the brachial plexus.

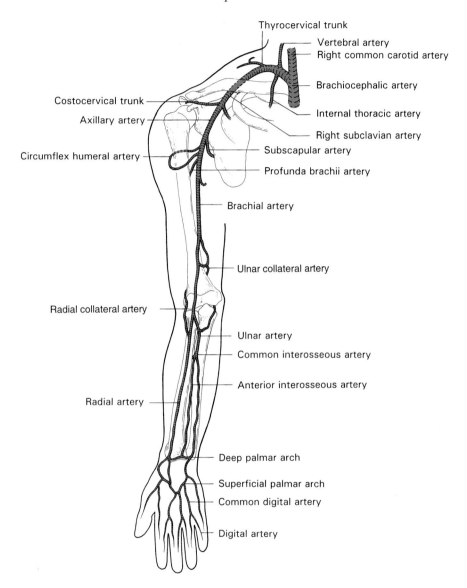

Fig. 2.18
The major arteries of the upper limb.

BRANCHES OF THE AXILLARY ARTERY

	Area of arterial supply
1. **Superior thoracic**	Pectorals and thoracic wall
2. **Thoraco-acromial**	Pectorals, breast, deltoid, acromion, sternoclavicular joint, subclavius
3. **Lateral thoracic**	Breast, serratus anterior, pectorals, subscapularis
4. **Subscapular**	Chest wall, muscles of back
5. **Anterior and posterior circumflex humeral**	Shoulder joint, humerus, muscles of shoulder region

The **brachial artery** is the continuation of the axillary artery and extends from the lower border of the teres major muscle to its termination in the lower regions of the cubital fossa. It bifurcates into the radial and ulnar arteries. The brachial artery lies on the medial aspect of the arm before passing more towards the midline as it pierces the bicipital aponeurosis.

BRANCHES OF THE BRACHIAL ARTERY

	Area of arterial supply
1. **Profunda brachee**	Muscles of arm, humerus elbow joint, skin of arm
2. **Nutrient**	Humerus
3. **Superior and inferior ulnar collateral**	Muscles of arm and around elbow, elbow joint

From the bifurcation of the brachial artery, the **radial artery** descends through the forearm lying on the radius and along the medial border of the brachioradialis muscle. It winds around the lateral aspect of the wrist to pass through the anatomical snuff box before terminating in the deep palmar arch.

BRANCHES OF THE RADIAL ARTERY

	Area of arterial supply
1. **Radial recurrent**	Elbow joint and muscles on radial side of elbow
2. **Muscular branches**	Muscles on posterior and radial aspect of forearm
3. **Carpal branches**	Carpals, wrist joint
4. **Superficial and deep palmar arch**	Metacarpals, digits, muscles on radial aspect
5. **Metacarpal branches**	Metacarpals, wrist joint, digits, muscles in hand

The **ulnar artery** accompanies the ulnar nerve through the medial aspect of the forearm and at the wrist it crosses superficial to the flexor retinaculum before terminating in the superficial palmar arch. Throughout its course it gives off the relatively large common interosseous branch which in turn bifurcates at the upper border of the interosseous membrane into the anterior and posterior interosseous arteries. The **anterior interosseous artery** passes through the anterior compartment of the forearm in the company of the anterior interosseous nerve. At the upper border of the pronator quadratus muscle it pierces the interosseous membrane to take part in the anastomosis around the wrist joint. The **posterior interosseous artery** passes down through the posterior compartment of the forearm and anastomoses with the anterior interosseous artery at the wrist.

BRANCHES OF THE ULNAR ARTERY

	Area of arterial supply
1. **Anterior and posterior ulnar recurrent.**	Elbow joint and muscles on ulnar side of elbow
2. **Common interosseous**	Deep muscles of forearm, radius, ulna, elbow joint
3. **Muscular branches**	Muscles on ulnar aspect of forearm
4. **Carpal branches**	Carpals, metacarpals, digits
5. **Superficial and deep palmar arch**	Muscles in hand, metacarpals, digits, wrist joint

The iliac arteries (Fig. 2.19) A, B

At the level of the fourth lumbar vertebra, the abdominal aorta terminates as the right and left **common iliac arteries**. The external iliac is generally recognized to be the continuation of the common iliac, and the internal iliac arises at the level of the disc between the fifth lumbar vertebra and the sacrum, anterior to the sacroiliac joint. There are generally no branches from the common iliac arteries. The **external iliac** is larger than the internal and it travels downwards, forwards and laterally to reach the midpoint of the inguinal ligament. Here it passes deep to the ligament and enters the thigh as the femoral artery. From its origin, the **internal iliac** runs inferiorly, to end opposite the upper border of the greater sciatic notch by dividing into anterior and posterior trunks. The branches of the anterior trunk supply the body wall, external genitalia, lower limb and pelvic viscera, while the posterior trunk is smaller and supplies only the body wall and the gluteal region.

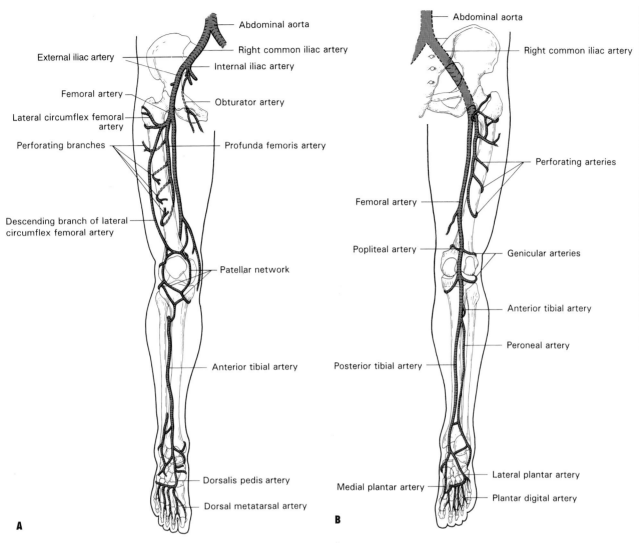

Fig. 2.19
The major arteries of the lower limb.

BRANCHES OF THE EXTERNAL ILIAC ARTERY

1. **Branches to the psoas major**

2. **Inferior epigastric** — Spermatic cord, anterior abdominal wall, peritoneum

3. **Deep circumflex iliac** — Abdominal musculature

BRANCHES OF THE INTERNAL ILIAC ARTERY

Anterior trunk	Area of arterial supply
1. **Superior and inferior vesical**	Bladder, ureter, prostate, seminal vesicles
2. **Middle and inferior rectal**	Lower rectum, anal canal, skin of buttock
3. **Uterine**	Ureter, cervix, vagina, uterus, uterine tubes
4. **Vaginal**	Vagina, bladder, rectum
5. **Penile branches**	Erectile tissue, penile skin
6. **Obturator**	Ilium, bladder, adductors of the thigh, muscles of ischial tuberosity, hip joint
7. **Internal pudendal**	External genitalia, muscles of pelvis and gluteal region
8. **Perineal**	Anus, penile bulb, scrotum, perineal muscles
9. **Inferior gluteal**	Buttock and back of thigh

Posterior trunk	
1. **Iliolumbar**	Cauda equina, muscles of posterior abdominal wall
2. **Lateral sacral**	Sacrum, cauda equina, skin and muscles over sacrum
3. **Superior gluteal**	Piriformis, obturator internus, innominate, skin and muscles of gluteal region

The arteries of the lower limb

(Fig. 2.19) A, B

The **femoral artery** is the continuation of the external iliac after it has passed under the inguinal ligament.

The femoral artery passes through the femoral triangle lateral to the femoral vein, enters the adductor canal and gains access to the popliteal fossa through the adductor hiatus where it lies anterior to the vein and the saphenous nerve crosses it from lateral to medial.

BRANCHES OF THE FEMORAL ARTERY

	Named branch	Area of arterial supply
1. **Superficial epigastric**		Anterior abdominal wall
2. **Superficial circumflex iliac**		Skin
3. **Superficial and deep external pudendal**		Skin of scrotum, lower abdomen
4. **Profunda femoris**	(1) Medial and lateral circumflex femoral	Femur, muscles around hip joint, hip joint
	(2) Perforating arteries	Muscles of thigh, femur
5. **Descending genicular**		Muscles around knee joint, knee joint, skin

The **popliteal artery** is the continuation of the femoral artery and passes from the tendinous arch of adductor magnus above to the lower border of the popliteus muscle, where it divides into the anterior and posterior tibial arteries.

The **anterior tibial artery** pierces the interosseous membrane, descends on its anterior surface and crosses the ankle midway between the malleoli. Here it becomes the dorsalis pedis artery and is the main

BRANCHES OF THE ANTERIOR TIBIAL ARTERY

	Area of arterial supply
1. **Anterior and posterior tibial recurrent**	Muscles around knee, knee joint, superior tibiofibular joint
2. **Muscular Branches**	Muscles throughout the anterior compartment of the leg
3. **Anterior medial and lateral malleolar**	Lower muscles of the leg, ankle joint
4. **Dorsalis pedis**	Ankle joint, bones of the foot and dorsal structures

arterial supply to the dorsum of the foot.

The **posterior tibial artery** descends through the posterior compartment of the leg in the company of the tibial nerve. It enters the foot by passing between the medial malleolus and the medial tubercle of the calcaneus. Here it divides into the medial and lateral plantar arteries, which are the principal arterial supply to the sole of the foot.

BRANCHES OF THE POSTERIOR TIBIAL ARTERY

	Area of arterial supply
1. **Circumflex fibular**	Neck of fibula, superior tibiofibular joint
2. **Peroneal**	Lateral compartment of leg, fibula, tarsals
3. **Branches to**	Tibia, muscles of posterior compartment of leg, ankle joint, heel
4. **Medial and lateral plantar**	Structures of plantar aspect of foot, heel, bones of foot

MAJOR VEINS

Veins of the head and neck (Fig. 2.13)

The majority of the **cardiac veins** drain into the coronary sinus. This runs in the posterior part of the left atrioventricular groove and terminates in the right atrium of the heart between the opening for the inferior vena cava and the tricuspid valve. Its tributaries are the great cardiac vein (which drains the left atrium and both ventricles), the small cardiac vein (which drains the right atrium and ventricle) and the middle cardiac vein (which drains both ventricles). The anterior cardiac veins drain the anterior aspect of the right ventricle and terminate in the right atrium. The venae cordis minimae open directly into the right atrium and ventricle, although they may also be found draining into the left atrium.

Veins of the head and neck (Fig. 2.20)

The **facial vein** forms at the angle of the eye by the union of the supratrochlear and supra-orbital veins. It passes obliquely downwards and runs deep to the zygomaticus major, risorius and platysma muscles before crossing the body of the mandible. In front of the angle of the mandible it is joined by the anterior division of the **retromandibular vein** and passes into the internal jugular vein near the greater cornu of the hyoid bone.

The **superficial temporal vein** drains the network in the scalp and unites in the substance of the parotid gland with the **maxillary vein** to form the **retromandibular vein**. This divides into an anterior and a posterior division, the former uniting with the facial vein and the latter uniting with the **posterior auricular vein** to form the **external jugular vein**.

The **external jugular vein** (Fig. 2.20) receives venous blood from the scalp and face. It is formed from the union of the posterior division of the retromandibular vein and the posterior auricular vein. It runs from the angle of the mandible to the middle of the clavicle and crosses the sternocleidomastoid muscle before terminating in the **subclavian vein**. The **internal jugular vein** is the continuation of the sigmoid sinus, extending from the jugular foramen and passing downwards through the neck in the carotid sheath in the company of the carotid arteries and the vagus nerve. It passes behind the sternal end of the clavicle and unites with the **subclavian vein** to form the **brachiocephalic vein**.

Veins of the upper limb (Fig. 2.21)

The **cephalic vein** originates from the dorsal venous network of the hand and passes around the radial

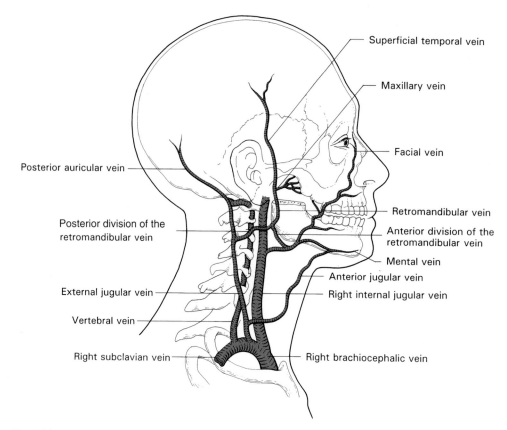

Fig. 2.20
The major veins of the head and neck.

aspect of the forearm. Before it passes in front of the elbow it receives the **median cubital** tributary. The cephalic vein then ascends lateral to the biceps brachii muscle, passes through the deltopectoral triangle and terminates in the **axillary vein**.

The **basilic vein** also drains the dorsal venous network of the hand and ascends through the forearm along its ulnar aspect. It is generally joined by the median cubital branch of the cephalic vein before ascending through the arm on the lateral aspect of the biceps brachii muscle. It continues as the axillary vein at the lower border of the teres major muscle.

The **median vein of the forearm** (median antebrachial vein) drains the palmar venous plexus and ascends in a virtually midline position up the anterior aspect of the forearm, where it may end in either the basilic or the median cubital vein.

The **axillary** vein commences at the lower border of the teres major muscle and ends at the outer border of the first rib where it continues as the **subclavian vein**. This latter vein passes to the medial border of the scalenus anterior muscle where it unites with the internal jugular vein to form the **brachiocephalic vein**.

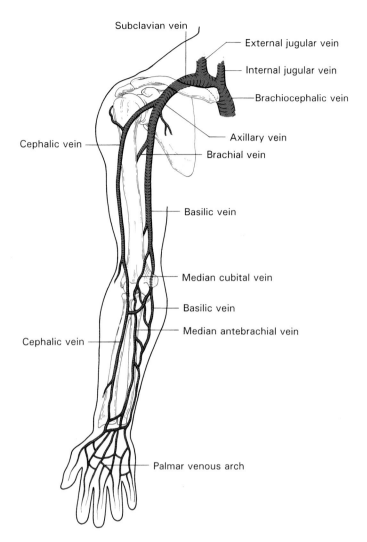

Subclavian vein

External jugular vein

Internal jugular vein

Brachiocephalic vein

Cephalic vein

Axillary vein

Brachial vein

Basilic vein

Median cubital vein

Basilic vein

Median antebrachial vein

Cephalic vein

Palmar venous arch

Fig. 2.21
The major veins of the upper limb.

Veins of the thorax (Fig. 2.22)

The **brachiocephalic vein** is formed from the union of the internal jugular and subclavian veins behind the sternal end of the clavicle. The left brachiocephalic vein is substantially longer than the right and they fuse behind the lower border of the right first costal cartilage and give rise to the **superior vena cava**. The tributaries of the brachiocephalic vein are the vertebral, internal thoracic,

inferior thyroid, superior intercostal and posterior intercostal veins. The **superior vena cava** collects venous blood from the area of the body superior to the diaphragm and conveys it to the right atrium of the heart. It commences behind the lower border of the first right costal cartilage and descends vertically behind the first and second intercostal spaces. Apart from the brachiocephalic veins, its only real tributaries arise from the azygos venous network.

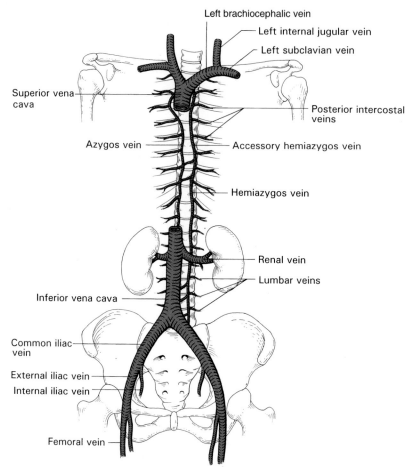

Left brachiocephalic vein
Left internal jugular vein
Left subclavian vein
Superior vena cava
Posterior intercostal veins
Azygos vein
Accessory hemiazygos vein
Hemiazygos vein
Renal vein
Lumbar veins
Inferior vena cava
Common iliac vein
External iliac vein
Internal iliac vein
Femoral vein

Fig. 2.22
The major veins of the trunk.

Veins of the lower limb (Fig. 2.23) A, B

The **great saphenous vein** passes from the medial margin of the foot and courses in front of the medial malleolus before ascending to the knee. It runs posteromedial to the medial condyles of the tibia and femur and ascends through the thigh to the saphenous opening where it drains into the **femoral vein**. The **small saphenous vein** passes behind the lateral malleolus and ascends through the middle of the back of the leg lateral to the tendo calcaneus. It then runs between the two heads of the gastrocnemius muscle and ends in the **popliteal vein**. The **posterior tibial** veins follow the same course as the posterior tibial artery through the posterior compartment of the leg, and unite with the **anterior tibial veins** (which run with the anterior interosseous artery) to form the **popliteal** vein. The **popliteal** vein then traverses the adductor hiatus and becomes the **femoral vein** as it ascends through the adductor canal and the femoral triangle. As the vein passes under the inguinal ligament it becomes the **external iliac vein**.

Veins of the abdomen and pelvis
(Fig. 2.22)

The **external iliac vein** is the continuation of the femoral vein, and it passes around the pelvic brim, anterior to the sacro-iliac joint where it is joined by the **internal iliac vein** to form the **common iliac vein**. The tributaries of the external iliac vein are the inferior epigastric, deep circumflex iliac and pubic veins. The tributaries of the internal iliac vein are the gluteal, internal pudendal, obturator, lateral sacral, middle rectal, vesical, uterine and vaginal veins. The right and left **common iliac** veins terminate at the right-hand side of the fifth lumbar vertebra by uniting to form the **inferior vena cava**. Thus, the inferior vena cava conveys venous blood from all aspects of the body inferior to the diaphragm, towards the right atrium of the heart. It ascends along the right-hand side of the vertebral column and occupies a deep groove on the posterior aspect of the liver before piercing the tendinous part of the diaphragm and opening into the right atrium. The tributaries of the inferior vena cava

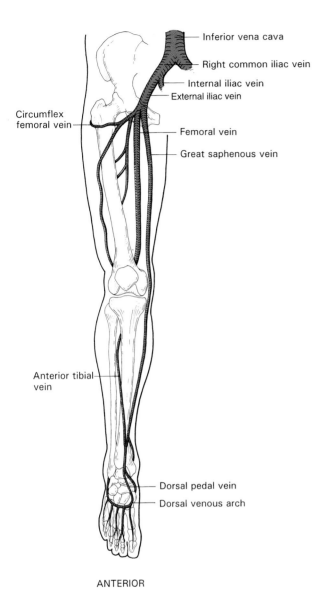

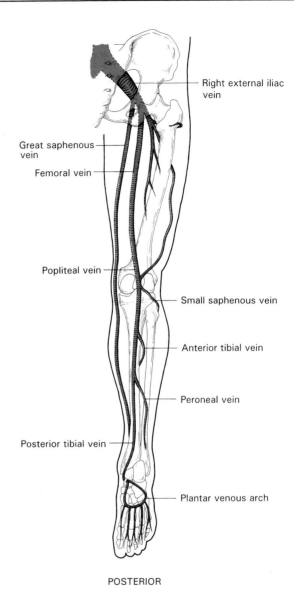

ANTERIOR

POSTERIOR

Fig. 2.23
The major veins of the lower limb.

are the lumbar, right testicular/ovarian, renal, right suprarenal, inferior phrenic and hepatic veins.

HEPATIC PORTAL SYSTEM (Fig. 2.24)

The venous blood from the region of gut between the lower esophagus and the upper part of the anal canal eventually drains into the **hepatic portal vein**, which is formed from the union of the **splenic vein** with the **superior mesenteric vein**. The hepatic portal vein is

formed at the level of the second lumbar vertebra and passes in front of the inferior vena cava and behind the neck of the pancreas. It ascends in the right border of the lesser omentum in front of the epiploic foramen to reach the porta hepatis. The tributaries of the splenic vein are the short gastric, left gastro-epiploic, pancreatic and inferior mesenteric veins. The tributaries of the superior mesenteric vein are the jejunal, ileal, ileocolic, right colic, middle colic, right gastro-epiploic and pancreaticoduodenal veins.

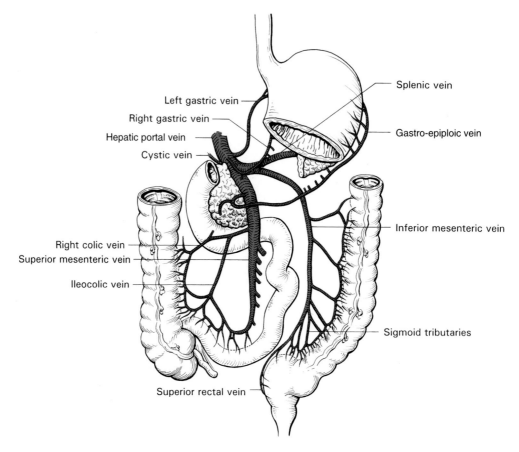

Fig. 2.24
The major tributaries of the hepatic portal venous system.

EMBRYONIC DEVELOPMENT OF THE HEART

The heart forms at the cranial end of the embryonic disc in an area called the cardiogenic region. Around day 19 of intra-uterine life, a pair of lateral endocardial tubes develops in response to signals from the underlying endoderm (Fig. 2.25A). During week 3, when embryonic folding occurs, these tubes are brought together in the midline and fuse to form a single primitive heart tube (Fig. 2.25B). By day 21 the heart has undergone a series of foldings, remodeling and septation to transform its single cavity into 4 chambers (Figs 2.25C–D). Transient chambers are initially formed – sinus venosus, primitive atrium, ventricle and bulbus cordis. The bulbus cordis develops into the right ventricle, the primitive ventricle gives rise to most of the left ventricle, whilst the superior end of the bulbus cordis forms the conus cordis and truncus arteriosus. The left sinus horn becomes the coronary sinus and the right sinus horn is incorporated into the wall of the right atrium. During weeks 5–6 the septum primum and the septum secundum of the interatrial wall begin to develop (Fig. 2.25E), as do both the tricuspid and mitral valves.

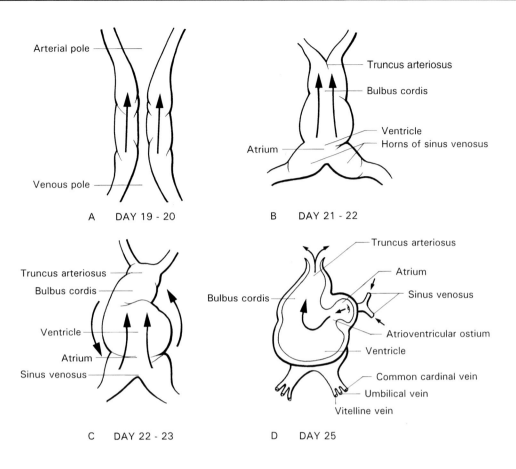

A   DAY 19 - 20

Arterial pole

Venous pole

B   DAY 21 - 22

Truncus arteriosus

Bulbus cordis

Ventricle

Horns of sinus venosus

Atrium

C   DAY 22 - 23

Truncus arteriosus

Bulbus cordis

Ventricle

Atrium

Sinus venosus

D   DAY 25

Truncus arteriosus

Atrium

Sinus venosus

Bulbus cordis

Atrioventricular ostium

Ventricle

Common cardinal vein

Umbilical vein

Vitelline vein

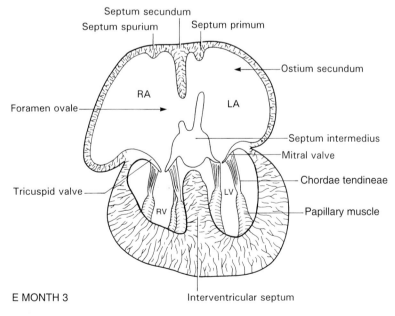

Septum secundum

Septum spurium

Septum primum

Ostium secundum

RA

LA

Foramen ovale

Septum intermedius

Mitral valve

Chordae tendineae

Tricuspid valve

Papillary muscle

RV

LV

E MONTH 3

Interventricular septum

Fig. 2.25
The embryonic development of the heart.

68 FETAL CIRCULATION

In the fetus, oxygenated blood enters the body via the left umbilical vein (Fig. 2.26). It mixes with deoxygenated portal blood in the ductus venosus and enters the inferior vena cava where it mixes with deoxygenated blood returning from the trunk and lower limbs. This mixed blood passes to the right atrium, where the orientation of the opening of the inferior vena cava ensures that much of the blood bypasses the right ventricle by passing directly to the left atrium via the foramen ovale. Some of the blood that does enter the right ventricle, mainly from the superior vena cava and the coronary sinus, will pass to the lung tissue, but much will be diverted from the pulmonary trunk to the aorta via the ductus arteriosus. In the left atrium, oxygenated blood from the right atrium mixes with blood returning from the lungs, and this is transferred to the left ventricle before being expelled into the aorta for distribution to the head, neck, upper limbs and ultimately the trunk and lower limbs.

The transition from total maternal dependence to virtual independence at birth brings about dramatic changes in the pattern of blood circulation within the newborn. As the alveoli fill with air following the first inspiration, the constricted pulmonary vessels open and the resistance of the pulmonary vasculature dramatically plummets. At the same time, obstetrical clamping of the umbilical vessels cuts off the flow from the placenta. The opening of the pulmonary circulation and the cessation of umbilical flow create changes in pressure and flow that cause the ductus arteriosus to constrict and the foramen ovale to close. Constriction of the ductus arteriosus will occur within 10–15 h of birth, as will constriction of the ductus venosus (ligamentum venosum). A patent ductus arteriosus (PDA) arises when closure is not completed and this results in the presence of a large shunt vessel. The initial closing of the foramen ovale is a mechanical phenomenon caused by the reversal in pressure between the two atria. The opening of the pulmonary vasculature and the cessation of umbilical flow reduce the pressure in the right atrium, whereas the sudden increase in pulmonary venous return raises the pressure in the left atrium. This pressure change forces the septum primum against the septum secundum thereby functionally closing the foramen ovale. However,

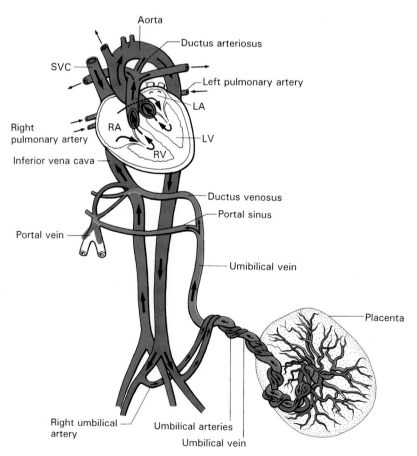

Fig. 2.26
A summary of the fetal circulation.

tissue fusion will not be complete until 3 months following birth and will leave a shallow depression on the interatrial wall – the fossa ovalis.

PULSE

When an artery lies close to the surface of the skin, a pulse can be felt which reflects the beating speed of the heart, or more specifically the contraction rate of the left ventricle. Figure 2.27 shows the location of the major arterial pulse points. Venous pulses can be detected in larger veins and this occurs as a result of the changes in pressure that accompany atrial contractions.

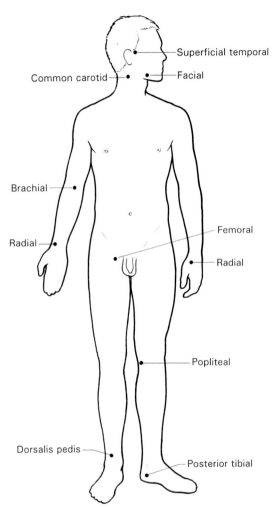

Superficial temporal

Facial

Common carotid

Brachial

Femoral

Radial

Radial

Popliteal

Dorsalis pedis

Posterior tibial

Fig. 2.27
A summary of the important pulse points.

PULSE POINTS

Artery	Location of pulse
Superficial temporal	Anterior to the ear at the root of the zygomatic process
Facial	At the inferior border of the mandible
Common carotid	Anterolateral aspect of the neck in the groove between the trachea and the strap muscles. Anterior to the sternocleidomastoid
Brachial	Anterior to the elbow joint (deep palpation)
Radial	Anterior to the distal radius. Lateral to the flexor carpi radialis tendon. Can also be felt in the anatomical snuffbox
Femoral	2–3 cm inferior to midpoint of the inguinal ligament in the femoral triangle
Popliteal	In popliteal fossa with the knee joint slightly flexed (deep palpation)
Dorsalis pedis	Dorsum of the foot. Lateral to the flexor hallucis longus tendon
Posterior tibial	Halfway between the medial malleolus and the tendo calcaneus

3

The nervous system

The nervous system can be separated either functionally into somatic and autonomic divisions, or anatomically into central and peripheral components (Fig. 3.1).

The **somatic** nervous system is essentially under voluntary or conscious control and:

a. provides motor supply to the striped muscles of the head and neck, body wall, limbs and diaphragm, and
b. receives sensory information both from external sources (exteroceptive) and internal body structures (proprioceptive).

It can be subdivided further into a **central** and a **peripheral** somatic nervous system. The central nervous system (CNS) comprises the brain and spinal cord and both are housed within a protective bony structure, covered by meninges and bathed in cerebrospinal fluid (CSF). The peripheral nervous system (PNS) comprises those processes that extend outwards from the CNS conveying both motor (efferent) and sensory (afferent) information to and from a peripheral site. The peripheral processes of the brain are the 12 pairs of cranial nerves and those of the spinal cord are the 31 pairs of spinal nerves.

The **autonomic** nervous system is essentially involuntary and operates below conscious level, supplying smooth muscle and viscera. Although the autonomic nervous system carries both motor and sensory information, it is fundamentally subdivided into sympathetic and parasympathetic divisions on the basis of the antagonistic action of its motor components. The motor fibers of the **sympathetic** division exit from the spinal cord in the thoracolumbar region and pass to the sympathetic chains which lie in the paravertebral gutters. From here, sympathetic nerves pass to the effector tissues and are responsible for preparing the body for emergencies by increasing the heart rate, initiating peripheral vasoconstriction, contraction of the smooth muscle of the body sphincters, pupillary constriction, etc. The **parasympathetic** efferent component is antagonistic in action and has a craniosacral outflow passing in the third, seventh, ninth and tenth cranial nerves as well as in the spinal nerves of the second to fourth sacral segments. It is involved in relaxing the body by decreasing the heart rate, initiating peripheral vasodilation, relaxation of sphincters, pupillary dilation, etc. The autonomic components also convey sensory information from viscera. Conscious sensory information is appreciated in terms of diffuse pain and an awareness of visceral distension. Subconscious afferent information is conveyed by baroreceptors and chemoreceptors that monitor changes in blood pressure and chemical composition.

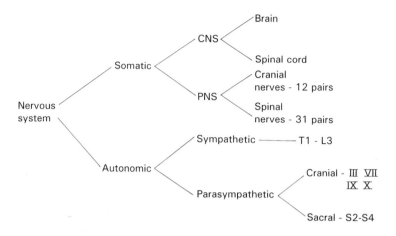

Fig. 3.1
Divisions of the nervous system.

NEUROEMBRYOLOGY

The trilaminar embryonic disc is the precursor of all fetal tissue derivatives and is formed by day 16 of fetal life (Fig. 3.2). At this stage a thickening is seen in the ectoderm along the mid-sagittal axis forming the neural plate. During week 4, this plate folds in a craniocaudal direction to form the **neural groove**. As the lateral lips of the developing tube come together they give rise to the **neural crest cells** which will eventually migrate and differentiate into many diverse structures, e.g. odontoblasts, some cranial nerve ganglia, the dermis and hypodermis of the face and neck, pharyngeal arch cartilages, connective tissue

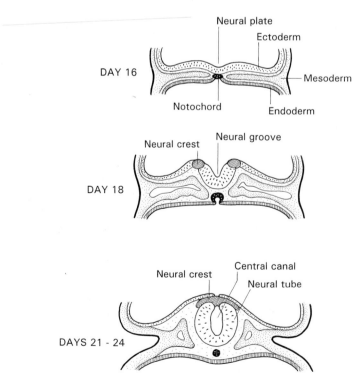

Fig. 3.2
The early embryological development of the nervous system.

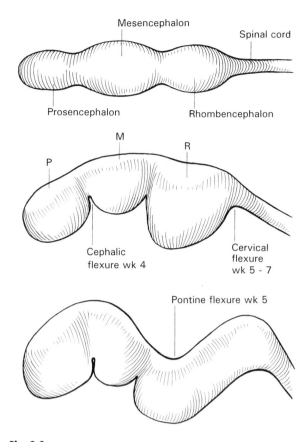

Fig. 3.3
Differentiation of the cranial pole of the neural tube.

surrounding the eye, pupillary and ciliary muscles, pre-aortic ganglia, adrenal medulla, dorsal root ganglia, chain ganglia, Schwann cells, glial cells in peripheral ganglia, arachnoid and pia mater, melanocytes, enteric ganglia etc.

By the beginning of week 4, the neural tube has started to show differentiation in the cranial region into the 3 primary brain vesicles (Fig. 3.3) forming the precursors of the forebrain, midbrain and hindbrain (prosencephalon, mesencephalon and rhombencephalon respectively). At around day 22, the cephalic end of the tube bends sharply forwards forming the mesencephalic flexure and during weeks 5–7 a second (cervical) flexure develops at the junction between the rhombencephalon and the spinal cord. Also in week 5 a third (pontine) flexure develops which causes a backwards bending in the region of the rhombencephalon. Therefore, by week 7 and following significant bilateral development of the prosencephalon, the 5 secondary brain vesicles have developed (Fig. 3.4). The central canal of the neural tube expands into these vesicles forming the ventricles of the brain. Thus, by the end of the second fetal month, the precursors of the brain and spinal cord, are well formed (Fig. 3.5).

At the end of week 4, neuroblasts in the spinal cord become organized into 4 columns – paired ventral (basal) and paired dorsal (alar) columns, which are

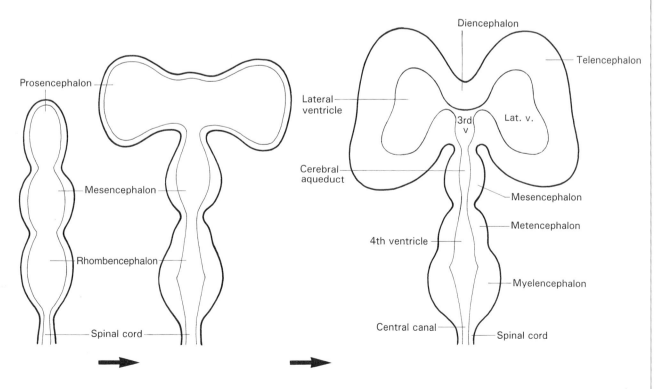

Fig. 3.4
Differentiation of the brain vesicles.

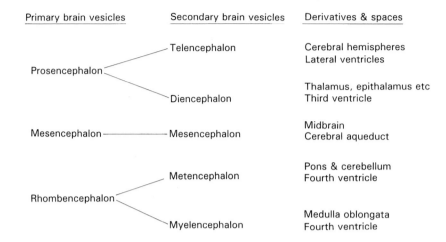

Primary brain vesicles	Secondary brain vesicles	Derivatives & spaces
Prosencephalon	Telencephalon	Cerebral hemispheres Lateral ventricles
	Diencephalon	Thalamus, epithalamus etc Third ventricle
Mesencephalon	Mesencephalon	Midbrain Cerebral aqueduct
Rhombencephalon	Metencephalon	Pons & cerebellum Fourth ventricle
	Myelencephalon	Medulla oblongata Fourth ventricle

Fig. 3.5
Derivatives of the primary brain vesicles.

separated by a lateral sulcus limitans (Fig. 3.6). The **ventral** columns will eventually develop into somatic motor neurons. The cells of the **dorsal** columns will develop into association neurons which connect the motor neurons of the central columns with neuronal processes that grow into the cord from the sensory neurons of the dorsal root ganglia which have developed from migrated neural crest cells. Somatic motor axons initially emerge from the ventral columns of the spinal cord at around day 30 of fetal development and grow towards the sclerotomes. As the motor root approaches the dorsal root ganglion it is stimulated to produce branching axon sprouts that pass either medially towards the spinal column or laterally to join up with the motor root and so form the spinal nerve. A spinal nerve is, therefore, a nerve of mixed motor and sensory axons that forms at each spinal level by the confluence of the dorsal and ventral root derivatives.

The motor and sensory innervation to the body wall and limbs is highly organized, not only in a segmental pattern (dermatomes and myotomes) which is established by somite differentiation, but also in a topographical pattern with motor components occupying a ventral location and sensory components a dorsal location. The somatic innervation of the head and neck is more complex as the cranial nerves are not so strictly regimented in terms of their specific target location or in the functional composition of the individual nerve. However, the cranial nerves still tend to adopt a topographical location in terms of the origin of their fiber types. Sensory neurons tend to adopt a dorsal location as they travel to higher centers and their central nuclei are more laterally placed, whereas motor neurons tend to adopt a more ventral location as

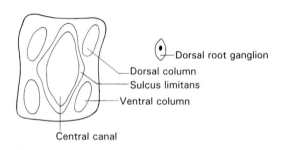

Dorsal root ganglion
Dorsal column
Sulcus limitans
Ventral column
Central canal

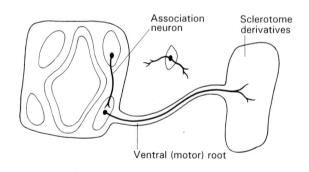

Association neuron
Sclerotome derivatives
Ventral (motor) root

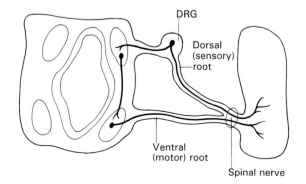

DRG
Dorsal (sensory) root
Ventral (motor) root
Spinal nerve

Fig. 3.6
Early embryonic development of the spinal nerves.

they descend to lower centers and their nuclei occupy a more medial position. The cranial nerve nuclei are organized into 7 distinct columns on the basis of their function (Fig. 3.7). The **general somatic efferent** column comprises the motor components of cranial nerves III, IV, VI and XII. The **general visceral efferent** column comprises the autonomic parasympathetic innervation via cranial nerves III (Edinger–Westphal nucleus), VII and IX (salivatory nuclei) and the dorsal nucleus of cranial nerve X. The **special visceral efferent** (branchiomotor) column comprises the motor components of cranial nerves V, VII, IX, X and XI. The sensory columns comprise the **general visceral afferent** neurons in cranial nerve X, the **special visceral afferents** in cranial nerves VII, IX and X subserving taste, the **general somatic afferent** fibers in cranial nerve V and the **special somatic afferent** column carrying both balance and hearing information via cranial nerve VIII.

THE SOMATIC NERVOUS SYSTEM AND RELATED STRUCTURES

The skull

The skull is comprised of an anterior facial or splanchnocranium and a more robust neurocranium

(Fig. 3.8) which offers protection to the brain. On removal of the calvarium (skull cap), it can be seen that the intracranial area is separated into 3 regions or cranial fossae (Fig. 3.9).

The **anterior cranial fossa** houses the frontal lobes of the brain and is bounded anteriorly by the frontal bone and posteriorly by the lesser wings of the sphenoid. The floor of the fossa is formed from the orbital plates of the frontal bone laterally and the cribriform plate of the ethmoid and jugum of the sphenoid bone in the midline. The ethmoid has a vertical projection, the crista galli, which passes upwards between the two cerebral hemispheres and serves as the site of attachment for the anterior extent of the falx cerebri. Anterior to the crista galli is the foramen caecum for the passage of an emissary vein from the nose to the superior sagittal sinus. The olfactory nerves pass from the roof of the nose through the cribriform plate to terminate in the olfactory bulb of the first cranial nerve. At the lateral and anterior margins of the cribriform plate is the anterior ethmoidal canal which is traversed by the anterior ethmoidal nerve and vessels passing from the orbit into the nose. The posterior ethmoidal canal is smaller and is for the passage of the posterior ethmoidal vessels. The lesser wings of the sphenoid pass backwards and medially and terminate in the anterior clinoid processes, which are the site of attachment of the free border of the tentorium cerebelli.

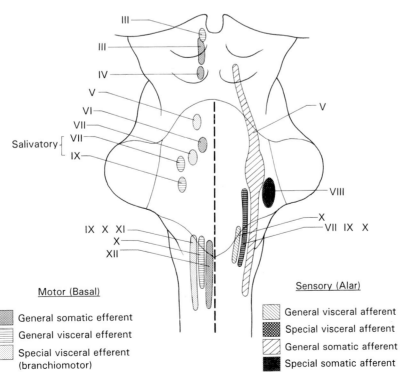

Fig. 3.7
Organization of the brainstem cranial nerve nuclei.

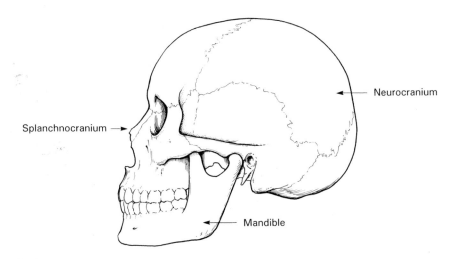

Fig. 3.8
Lateral view of the skull.

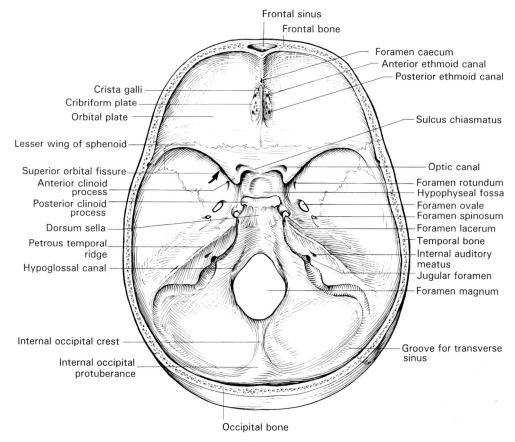

Fig. 3.9
The intracranial cavities.

The sphenoparietal sinuses run along the free border of the lesser wings of the sphenoid before terminating in the cavernous sinuses, lateral to the body of the sphenoid. Between the two anterior clinoid processes and posterior to the jugum of the sphenoid is a midline plateau of bone which connects the medial margins of the two optic canals. This is the sulcus chiasmatus on which the optic chiasma lies.

The **middle cranial fossa** houses the temporal lobes of the brain and is deeper than the anterior cranial fossa. It is bounded anteriorly by the greater and lesser wings of the sphenoid bone, laterally by the squamous parts of the temporal bones and posteriorly by the petrous temporal crests. The body of the sphenoid lies in the midline and it houses the pituitary gland in the hypophyseal fossa. The dorsum sella marks the posterior boundary of the hypophyseal fossa and terminates in 2 posterior clinoid processes, which are the site of attachment for the fixed border of the tentorium cerebelli. The middle cranial fossa communicates with the orbits via the optic canals and the superior orbital fissures. Each optic canal lies medial to the anterior clinoid process and is traversed by the optic nerve and the ophthalmic artery (a branch of the internal carotid artery). The internal carotid artery occupies a groove medial to the anterior clinoid process and inferior to the optic canal which can be converted into a bony caroticoclinoid canal by the fusion of the anterior and middle clinoid processes. The superior orbital fissure is the means whereby all other structures from the intracranial region enter or leave the orbit. These structures include branches of the ophthalmic nerve, the oculomotor, trochlear and abducens nerves, and the ophthalmic veins which pass backwards into the cavernous sinus. In the floor of the middle cranial fossa (greater wing of the sphenoid bone) is the foramen rotundum which leads forwards into the pterygopalatine fossa and transmits the maxillary division of the trigeminal nerve. Posterior to this is the foramen ovale, which also pierces the greater wing of the sphenoid and communicates below with the infratemporal fossa, transmitting the mandibular division of the trigeminal nerve and the lesser petrosal nerve. If an accessory meningeal artery is present then it will also pass through this foramen. The foramen spinosum lies posterolateral to the foramen ovale and transmits the middle meningeal vessels and the meningeal branch of the mandibular nerve. Posterior to the foramen ovale is the foramen lacerum, which forms at the junction of the sphenoid and temporal bones. The only structures to pass through this foramen are the meningeal branches of the ascending pharyngeal artery and some emissary veins. The internal carotid artery and its postganglionic sympathetic plexus travel across the intracranial opening before turning anteriorly to pass lateral to the body of the sphenoid. In the foramen, the deep petrosal nerve joins with the greater petrosal nerve to form the nerve of the pterygoid canal. Behind the foramen lacerum on the petrous temporal ridge is a shallow depression, the cavum trigeminale, occupied by the trigeminal sensory ganglion. Behind this is a groove for the superior petrosal venous sinus, which connects the cavernous to the sigmoid sinus.

The **posterior cranial fossa** is the largest and deepest of the three fossae. Its boundaries are the sphenoid, basi-occipital and temporal bones anteriorly and the squamous occipital bone laterally and posteriorly. On the posterior wall of the fossa is the internal occipital protuberance and the confluence of the sinuses with the deep grooves for the transverse venous sinuses passing laterally. The internal occipital crest is the site of attachment of the falx cerebelli, a double fold of dura mater that passes vertically between the cerebellar hemispheres. The posterior cranial fossa houses the occipital lobes of the cerebral hemispheres superiorly and the midbrain and the components of the hindbrain (the medulla oblongata, pons and cerebellum) inferiorly. The fossa is partitioned by the horizontally placed tentorium cerebelli except at the tentorial notch where the midbrain passes to connect with the forebrain in the middle cranial fossa. In the posterior wall of the petrous part of the temporal bone is the internal acoustic or auditory meatus. This transmits the facial and vestibulocochlear nerves and the labyrinthine vessels. Directly below this is the jugular foramen with its deep groove for the sigmoid sinus. This foramen transmits the sigmoid sinus (which becomes the internal jugular vein), the inferior petrosal sinus and the glossopharyngeal, vagus and accessory nerves. The hypoglossal canal lies at the anterolateral boundary of the foramen magnum and transmits the hypoglossal nerve and some of the meningeal branches of the ascending pharyngeal artery. The medulla oblongata and its covering meninges pass out through the foramen magnum in the floor of the fossa to become continuous with the spinal cord. Other structures passing through this foramen are the vertebral arteries with their spinal branches passing in the opposite direction and the spinal part of the accessory nerve.

MAJOR CRANIAL FORAMINA

Intracranial foramina

Foramen caecum	Emissary vein
Cribriform plate	Olfactory nerves, anterior ethmoid nerve and vessels and osterior ethmoid vessels
Optic canal	Optic nerve, meninges and ophthalmic artery
Superior orbital fissure	Ophthalmic nerve, oculomotor, trochlear and abducens nerves, ophthalmic veins, orbital branch of middle meningeal artery, postganglionic sympathetic nerves and recurrent meningeal branch of lacrimal artery
Foramen rotundum	Maxillary nerve
Foramen ovale	Mandibular nerve, lesser petrosal nerve and accessory meningeal artery
Foramen spinosum	Middle meningeal vessels and meningeal branch of mandibular nerve
Foramen lacerum	Meningeal branches of ascending pharyngeal artery and emissary veins
Pterygoid canal	Deep petrosal nerve, greater petrosal nerve and pterygoid artery
Internal acoustic meatus	Facial and vestibulocochlear nerves and labyrinthine vessels
Jugular foramen	Glossopharyngeal, vagus and accessory nerves, sigmoid venous sinus and inferior petrosal sinus
Hypoglossal canal	Hypoglossal nerve, meningeal branches of ascending pharyngeal artery and emissary veins
Foramen magnum	Medulla oblongata, meninges, vertebral arteries, spinal arteries, spinal branch of accessory nerve, apical ligament of dens and membrana tectoria

Foramina on base of skull

Carotid canal	Internal carotid artery and postganglionic sympathetic plexus
Stylomastoid foramen	Facial nerve and stylomastoid branch of posterior auricular artery

Foramina on face

Supra-orbital foramen	Supra-orbital nerve and vessels
Infra-orbital foramen	Infra-orbital nerve and vessels
Mental foramen	Mental nerve and vessels

Vertebral column

The vertebral column extends in the midline from the base of the skull above to the pelvis below and then beyond as the rudimentary tail (Fig. 3.10). Although the adult column represents some two-fifths of standing height, only three-quarters of its length is derived from the bony vertebrae. The remaining quarter of the column comprises intervening fibrocartilaginous intervertebral discs. Only a small degree of movement occurs between any two individual vertebrae but the cumulative effect results in a column of considerable flexibility that has sacrificed neither its stability nor its strength.

The column as a whole performs 3 major functions:

1. it is the means whereby body weight is transferred from the upper regions to the pelvic girdle and then to the ground via the lower limbs
2. it provides a large site of attachment for the muscles of posture and locomotion, and
3. it offers a protective canal for the spinal cord and its covering meninges.

There are normally 24 true or presacral vertebrae which constitute the cervical, thoracic and lumbar regions of the column. The 7 cervical vertebrae extend from the base of the skull above to articulate with the first thoracic vertebra below at the root of the neck.

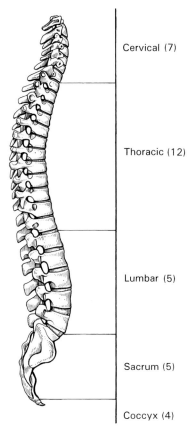

Fig. 3.10
Lateral view of the vertebral column.

This is arguably the most mobile region of the column and is the site of attachment for the strong vertebral muscles of the neck which are responsible for maintaining the erect position of the head. The cervical column houses the region of the spinal cord which carries the greatest proportion of white matter, so its protective function is vitally important. The first and second cervical vertebrae have been extensively modified from the general vertebral pattern to permit the movements of nodding and rotation of the head on the neck. The 12 thoracic vertebrae extend from the last cervical vertebra above to articulate with the first lumbar vertebra below. This region of the column is specialized for articulation with the ribs and is probably the least mobile segment of the presacral column. Not only are these vertebrae responsible for transferring axial body weight in a caudal direction but they also transfer upper lateral body weight via the ribs and pectoral girdle. The 5 lumbar vertebrae extend from the last thoracic vertebra above to articulate with the first sacral vertebra below at the lumbosacral angle. This region of the column is particularly well adapted to the transfer of body weight and also offers a large surface area for the muscles that are essential for the maintenance of upright posture of the trunk.

There are normally 9 false vertebrae, which make up the sacrum and the coccyx. In the adult, the sacrum is generally formed from 5 fused vertebrae which articulate superiorly with the last lumbar vertebra, inferiorly with the first coccygeal vertebra and laterally with the innominates at the sacroiliac joints. The large surface area of the sacrum allows the attachment of postural muscles as well as the muscles and ligaments of the gluteal region. The coccyx comprises a variable number of vertebrae, although there are normally 4. It is a vestigial structure which shows considerable variation in its morphology and composition. With advancing age, the coccyx may fuse to the sacrum particularly in the male.

The vertebral column is not a straight pillar of bone but consists of several curved segments which act like independent springs and so bestow considerable flexibility and resilience to the structure as a whole (Fig. 3.11). The curvatures are either primary or secondary, with the former being concave anteriorly and the latter convex anteriorly. In the fetus, the vertebral column is flexed in a 'C' shape with the

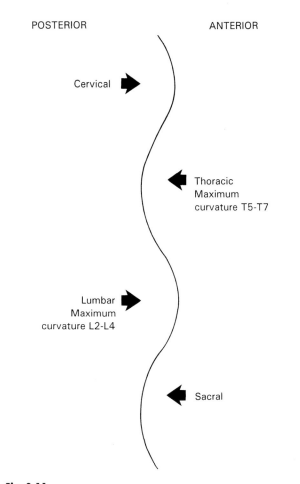

Fig. 3.11
The curvatures of the adult vertebral column.

concavity facing anteriorly and this shape is fundamentally maintained until birth. Once the child starts to hold its head up independently, at around 3–4 months, a compensatory secondary curve, which is convex anteriorly, develops in the cervical region. Once the child begins to sit up unaided, at around 6–8 months, a further secondary compensatory curve, which is also convex anteriorly, develops in the lumbar region. This secondary curve becomes progressively more pronounced as the child begins to walk.

The primary curves are maintained through the intrinsic shape of the bony vertebrae, whilst the secondary curves arise from a modification in shape of the cartilaginous intervertebral discs. With age, discs may degenerate and the integrity of the secondary curves become impaired. The column may then revert to its original primary curves which partly explains the curved shape of the vertebral column in the elderly. Given the developmental and functional origins of the secondary curves, it is perhaps not surprising to note that the majority of all back pain occurs in the compensatory regions of the neck and lumbar column.

Although the morphology of each vertebra is a product of localized factors and more general requirements that are placed on the column as a whole, a basic pattern can be identified in all adult vertebrae throughout the length of the column.

A typical vertebra (Fig. 3.12)

Viewed from above, the typical vertebra has an anterior body and a posterior neural arch which forms the boundaries of the vertebral foramen (spinal canal). The main function of the body is to transmit weight from the inferior surface of the vertebra above to the superior surface of the vertebra below via the intervertebral discs. As the column is descended, the bodies increase in size to accommodate the proportional increase in body weight that passes through them. Therefore, the lumbar vertebrae have the largest bodies and the cervical the smallest. The essentially flat superior and inferior surfaces of the body are the sites of attachment of the intervertebral discs that separate adjacent vertebrae and act as shock absorbers to dissipate the forces placed on the column

SUPERIOR VIEW

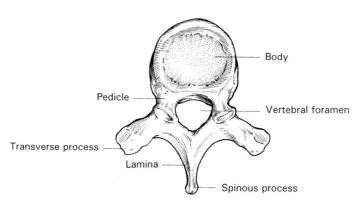

RIGHT LATERAL VIEW

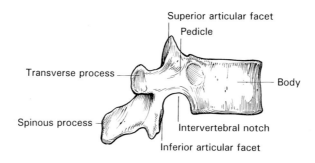

Fig. 3.12
A typical vertebra.

during locomotion. This is a secondary cartilaginous joint with a layer of hyaline cartilage covering the superior and inferior surfaces of the bodies, which are further separated by a fibrocartilaginous disc. This disc is composed of an outer annulus fibrosus and an inner nucleus pulposus, which is a remnant of the embryological notochord.

The neural arch of the vertebra is connected anteriorly to the body via 2 stout bars of bone called pedicles whose primary function is to transfer lateral body weight from the transverse processes to the midline vertebral body. The pedicles tend to be attached towards the superior poles of the bodies resulting in 2 notches of uneven depth when two vertebrae are articulated and viewed from the side. The inferior notch is usually deeper than the superior one, when two vertebrae articulate, an intervertebral foramen is formed through which pass the roots of the spinal nerves and the vascular structures supplying the spinal cord.

An articular pillar of paired superior and inferior articular processes lies behind the pedicles. The superior articular process of one vertebra articulates with the inferior articular process of the vertebra above via synovial joints. The superior articular facet is more ventrally placed with its articular surface facing posteriorly, whilst the inferior facet is more dorsally placed with the articular surface facing anteriorly. The superior articular facets are more closely related to the pedicles, whilst the inferior facets occur on the inner surface of the laminae of the neural arches.

The functions of the neural arch are to provide sites for muscle attachment and to offer a protective bony canal for the spinal cord and meninges. The neural arch has a single midline spinous process which projects posteriorly and paired transverse processes which pass laterally. The laminae of a typical vertebra connect the spinous to the transverse processes on each side and together they form a large surface area for muscle and ligament attachment.

There are 2 costal processes associated with each vertebra, which become particularly well developed in the thoracic region as ribs. However, virtually every vertebra bears some vestige of costal articulations.

Typical cervical vertebrae (Fig. 3.13)

A typical cervical vertebra is to be found in the middle of the segment, i.e. C3–C6, as C1 (atlas), C2 (axis) and C7 (vertebra prominens) are atypical. The typical cervical vertebra is characterized by a relatively small body that is wider in its transverse than in its anteroposterior dimension. Its superior surface is concave transversely and slightly convex in the anteroposterior plane. The lateral aspects of the superior surface are elevated into 2 lateral lips, or uncinate processes, which are the sites of the synovial

joints of Lushka. The transverse processes contain the foramen transversarium for the passage of the vertebral artery and its associated venous and postganglionic sympathetic plexuses. The anterior bar of the transverse process terminates in an anterior tubercle, which is connected to the posterior tubercle by an intertubercular lamella of bone, forming the shallow neural groove. Within each groove, the roots of the spinal nerve pass behind the position of the vertebral artery as it traverses the foramen transversarium. The anterior primary ramus of each spinal nerve crosses the groove, whilst the posterior ramus passes around the articular pillar to gain access to the muscles and skin of the back. The laminae are flat and long and increase in depth from C3 downwards. They terminate in a bifid spinous process which may be single in C6. The vertebral canal is somewhat triangular in cross-section and increases in size from C3 to C5, which corresponds with the thickest part of the cervical enlargement of the spinal cord that provides the innervation to the upper limb via the brachial plexus.

Atlas (Fig. 3.14)

The first cervical vertebra is atypical both in form and function. It is essentially a ring of bone that does not possess a true vertebral body. As such, the weight of the head is transmitted through the occipital condyles to the upper articular facets of the atlas and then through its inferior articular facets to the axis below. The atlas has robust anterior and posterior arches which are united by thick lateral masses that carry the upper and lower articular facets. The anterior arch bears a rounded articular facet on its posterior surface for the synovial articulation with the odontoid process (dens) of the axis. The dens is often considered to be the displaced body of the atlas, but this is certainly too simplistic a viewpoint. The superior surface of the posterior arch is grooved by the vertebral artery as it passes from the foramen transversarium towards the foramen magnum. It is accompanied in this position by the first cervical spinal nerve. A small spicule of bone (posterior ponticle), the ossified oblique ligament, may convert this groove into a foramen. The superior articular facets are kidney-shaped and deeply concave, being reciprocal in shape to the convex occipital condyles of the skull above. This shape permits extensive forward and backward nodding of the head as well as a considerable degree of lateral flexion. Rotation of the head in relation to the neck takes place at the articulation between the atlas and the dens. The lateral masses project into the spinal canal forming 2 spaces of unequal size. The anterior compartment is smaller and is occupied by the dens, which is held in position by the transverse ligament, which attaches to small tubercles on the inner surface of the lateral masses. The posterior compartment of the spinal canal, behind

SUPERIOR VIEW

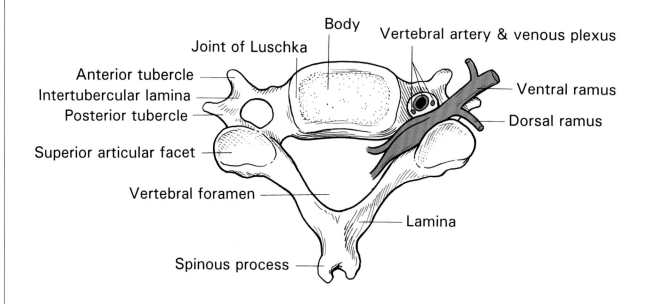

Body

Vertebral artery & venous plexus

Joint of Luschka

Anterior tubercle

Intertubercular lamina

Posterior tubercle

Ventral ramus

Dorsal ramus

Superior articular facet

Vertebral foramen

Lamina

Spinous process

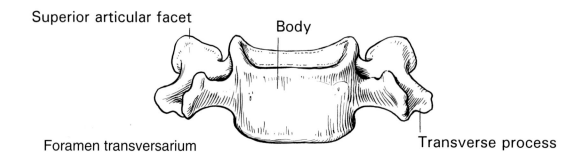

Superior articular facet

Body

Foramen transversarium

Transverse process

Fig. 3.13
A typical cervical vertebra.

the transverse ligament, houses the transitional zone between the lower limits of the medulla oblongata and the first cervical segment of the spinal cord. The transverse processes of the atlas are particularly long and are the sites of attachment for the muscles involved in rotation of the head. The apex of the transverse process bears a single tubercle, which can be palpated in the living, in the gap between the mastoid process and the angle of the mandible.

Axis (Fig. 3.15)
This vertebra is the pivot or axis upon which the head

turns and is readily identified by its projecting odontoid process or dens. C1 and C2 articulate via both the joint between the dens and the posterior surface of the anterior arch and the synovial superior and inferior articular processes. C2 articulates with C3 via the secondary cartilaginous articulation of the bodies and by the synovial joints, so that by the inferior surface of the axis the typical pattern of intervertebral articulation is established. The apex of the dens is attached to the occipital bone by apical ligaments and the slightly flattened posterolateral surface is the site of the attachment of the alar ligaments, which also pass

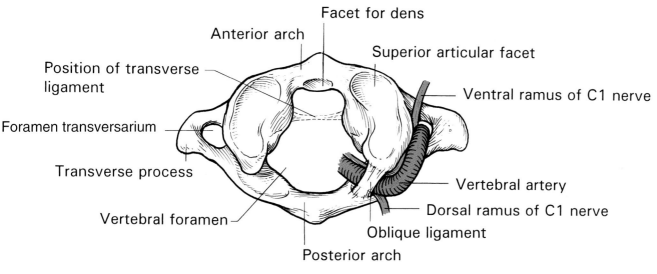

Fig. 3.14
The atlas (C1)

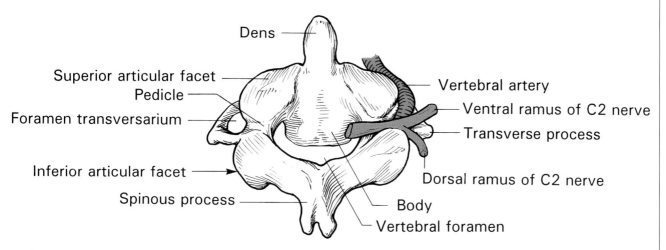

Fig. 3.15
The axis (C2).

superiorly. The dens is waisted by the passage of the transverse ligament, which helps to keep it securely in place. The true body of the axis is said to lie below the level of the dens. Unlike the remainder of the column, the superior and inferior articular facets of C2 do not take part in the vertical articular pillar. The superior facets are large, virtually horizontal, and round in shape for articulation with the atlas, whilst the inferior facets are much smaller, more vertically inclined and displaced more posteriorly. The laminae are particularly robust, fusing in a powerful bifid spinous process for the attachment of the muscles which extend, rotate and retract the head. The transverse processes are small and end in a single posterior tubercle. Each foramen transversarium is directed superolaterally, as the vertebral arteries deviate

laterally at this point to be in the correct position to pass through the corresponding foramen in the atlas. The anterior primary ramus of the second cervical spinal nerve passes lateral to the position of the vertebral artery.

Vertebra prominens
The seventh cervical vertebra is essentially transitional, adopting some characteristics of the cervical vertebrae above and others from the thoracic vertebrae below. It is called the vertebra prominens because of its particularly long spinous process which is visible under the skin and is not bifid. In reality, however, the spinous process of T1 may prove to be more prominent than that of C7. It usually possesses a foramen transversarium in its transverse process but, unlike the

more typical cervical vertebrae, it is only traversed by the venous and postganglionic sympathetic plexuses. In some instances, the anterior bar of the transverse process may remain separate, forming a cervical rib. These ribs are frequently asymptomatic but they can give rise to vascular complications due to stenosis of the subclavian artery or neurological disruptions due to compression on the lower roots of the brachial plexus.

Typical thoracic vertebrae

Thoracic vertebrae are characterized by the presence of articular facets on the bodies and transverse processes for articulation with the heads and tubercles respectively of the ribs. The description of a typical vertebra, as given on page 80, closely applies to most of the thoracic vertebrae. The bodies are somewhat heart-shaped when viewed from above, and have a small costal demi-facet on the lateral side of the body at the level of the superior border and a larger costal demi-facet in the same lateral location but on the inferior border. The superior demi-facet is the site of the synovial articulation with the lower facet on the head of the rib of the corresponding number, e.g. the second rib articulates with the superior demi-facet on T2. The inferior demi-facet is larger and articulates with the upper facet on the head of the rib that is one number lower in the series, e.g. the inferior demi-facet of T2

articulates with the head of the third rib. The inferior vertebral notches are deep and the superior are more shallow, so that the intervertebral notch is predominantly formed from the inferior boundaries of the vertebra above. The transverse processes are directed backwards and laterally, each carrying a costal facet on its anterior aspect for articulation with the tubercle of the rib of the same number. Generally the spinous processes are long, slender, point downwards and end in a single tubercle.

Atypical thoracic vertebrae (Fig. 3.16)

T1 is similar in its morphology to C7, with a body that is wider in its transverse than its anteroposterior dimensions. The upper costal facet (for articulation with the first rib) is complete and a small demi-facet is present on the lower border for the upper facet of the head of the second rib. In addition T1, and to a lesser extent T2, possess an upward-facing articular shelf in association with the superior articular facet. This shelf projects backwards and at virtually right angles to the lower margin of the superior articular facet, and acts as a stop to limit the downward displacement of the inferior articular surface of the vertebra above. These butting facets appear to permit a more even downward transmission of forces arising from muscles attached to the cervical transverse processes and, during excessive

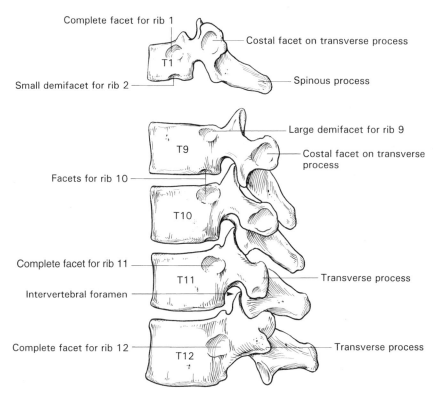

Fig. 3.16
Atypical thoracic vertebrae.

vertical compression, their impingement clearly absorbs some of the compressive force, thus giving relief to the vertebral bodies.

T9 may possess a costal demi-facet only on the superior part of the body and be devoid of one below, although there is always a corresponding articular facet present on the transverse process for the tubercle of the ninth rib. T10 has a whole costal articular facet above but does not possess an inferior one. A small articular facet may be present on the transverse process for the tenth rib. T11 and T12 are essentially transitional in shape between the thoracic vertebrae above and the lumbar vertebrae below. They are more robust and both have a single facet on the body for articulation with the rib of the corresponding number. The facet migrates posteriorly from the sides of the bodies to occupy a position on the sides of the pedicles. The transverse processes are reduced in size and no longer articulate with the ribs. The spinous processes are also reduced in length and are more horizontally aligned.

The spinal canal begins to widen again in the lower lumbar region to accommodate the lumbar spinal enlargement for the innervation of the lower limbs.

Lumbar vertebrae (Fig. 3.17)

These vertebrae are distinguished by their size and the lack of both foramina transversaria and costal articular facets. The bodies are large and kidney-shaped and the pedicles short and stout, indicating the importance of weight transfer in this region. The transverse processes are slender, the laminae are deep and short and the spinous processes are thick and square. The synovial superior and inferior articular processes are vertically oriented and curved transversely so that the lower pair are convex transversely and look forwards and laterally and are placed closer together than the upper pair which are concave transversely, wider apart and curve to look inwards and backwards. The spinal canal is triangular in shape. The body of L5 is somewhat wedge-shaped, being higher in the front than behind,

SUPERIOR VIEW

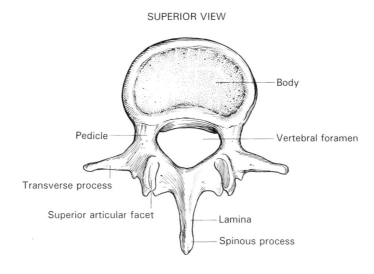

LEFT LATERAL VIEW

Fig. 3.17
A typical lumbar vertebra.

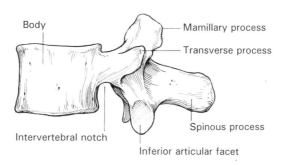

and so helps to form the characteristic lumbosacral angle.

Sacrum (Fig. 3.18)

In the adult, the 5 (or sometimes 6) vertebrae below the lumbar segment fuse to form the sacrum, which is the central axis of the pelvic girdle. This bony mass articulates superiorly with the last lumbar vertebra laterally with the innominates at the sacro-iliac joints and inferiorly with the first coccygeal segment. It is a wedge-shaped bone that is wider above at its base and narrower below at its apex. It is concave anteriorly both from above to below and from side to side, and convex posteriorly both from above to below and from side to side. On the ventral aspect it is clear that the central part is formed from the fusion of the sacral bodies, as the four transverse lines of fusion may persist even into old age. Lateral to this are 4 anterior sacral foramina, which are the remnants of the anterior boundaries of the intervertebral foramina, for the passage of the ventral rami of the sacral spinal nerves. The rounded bars of bone between adjacent foramina

are said to be the remnants of the heads and necks of ribs and are therefore costal in origin. Lateral to the foramina are the lateral masses, which are marked by neural grooves leading from the foramina and are also said to be costal in origin, although there is some debate over this statement. The lateral surfaces of the upper two lateral masses articulate with the auricular surface of each innominate, forming the sacro-iliac joints. The convex posterior surface represents the fused neural arches, with the midline sacral crest and spinous tubercles representing the fused spinous processes. Lateral to this is the intermediate (articular) crest which is formed from the fusion of the synovial articular pillar. Lateral to this are the 4 posterior sacral foramina, which are the remnants of the posterior boundaries of the intervertebral foramina, for the passage of the posterior rami of the sacral spinal nerves. Lateral to these is the lateral sacral crest, which is formed from the fusion of the transverse processes. In the lower part of the sacrum the laminae fail to meet; chey fuse in the midline, leaving a sacral hiatus bounded by the cornua of the sacrum. The sacral hiatus

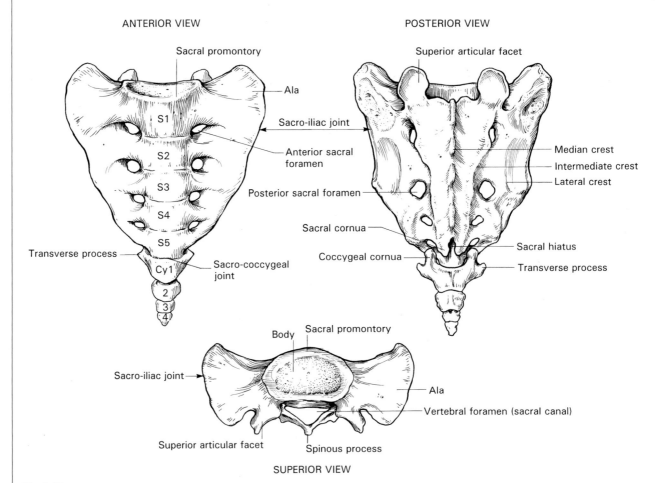

Fig. 3.18
The sacrum.

shows considerable variation in both length and width and this is important to bear in mind with regards to regional anaesthesia (Fig. 3.19). One of the methods of identification of the position of the hiatus relies on palpation of the posterior iliac spines of the innominate and the extrapolation to an equilateral triangle, where the apex will lie over the hiatus (Fig. 3.20).

Coccyx

This small region of the column comprises the fused 4 or 5 coccygeal vertebrae that make up the rudimentary tail (Fig. 3.18). The first segment usually carries vestiges of the transverse processes and upper articular facets (cornua), which are attached to the corresponding sacral cornua by ligaments. The upper surface of the superior coccygeal segment articulates with the apex of the sacrum and with advancing age this joint may synostose, more commonly in the male. The coccyx is the site of attachment for muscles of both the floor of the pelvis and the gluteal region.

Arthrology of the vertebral column

The important joints and ligaments of the vertebral column require some further discussion. Obviously, the joints of the occipito-atlanto-axial segment are unique, but the remainder of the arthrology is strikingly uniform.

The **atlanto-occipital joints** are synovial, with the convex surfaces of the occipital condyles articulating with the reciprocal concave facets of the superior articular surfaces of the atlas. The bones are united by the fibrous joint capsules and the anterior and posterior atlanto-occipital membranes (Figs 3.21 and 3.22). The **anterior atlanto-occipital membrane** is broad and dense and attached superiorly to the anterior margin of the foramen magnum. It extends inferiorly to attach to the upper border of the anterior arch of the atlas and is strengthened below by the anterior longitudinal ligament. The **posterior atlanto-occipital membrane** is thinner than its anterior counterpart and passes from the posterior margin of the foramen magnum above to the superior surface of the posterior arch of the atlas. It

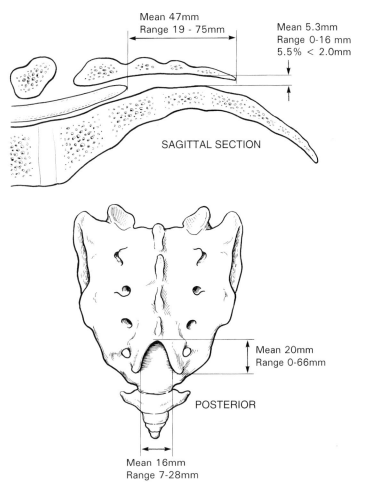

Mean 47mm
Range 19 - 75mm

Mean 5.3mm
Range 0-16 mm
5.5% < 2.0mm

SAGITTAL SECTION

Mean 20mm
Range 0-66mm

POSTERIOR

Mean 16mm
Range 7-28mm

Fig. 3.19
Dimensions of the sacral canal and hiatus.

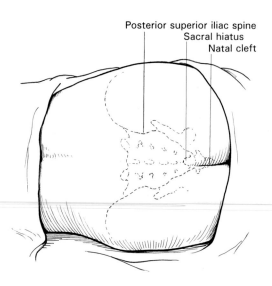

Fig. 3.20
The surface anatomy of the sacral hiatus.

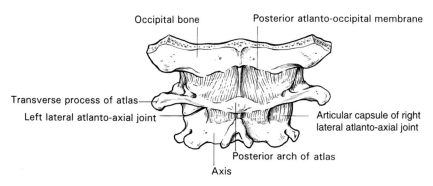

Fig. 3.21
Posterior view of the occipito-atlanto-axial joints.

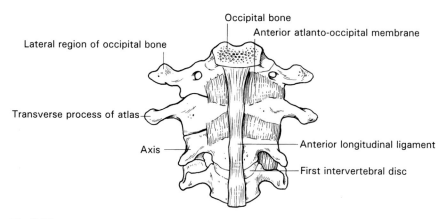

Fig. 3.22
Anterior view of the occipito-atlanto-axial region.

arches over the groove for the vertebral artery and so forms a canal for the artery and the first cervical spinal nerve. These joints can only operate in unison, never independently, with the range of possible movements being restricted to flexion and extension (nodding action) with a limited degree of lateral flexion.

The **atlanto-axial joints** are lateral (superior and inferior articular facets) and median (between the anterior arch of the atlas and the odontoid process of the axis). The pivotal action that occurs at the latter joint requires specialized muscular and ligamentous attachments; these include the transverse ligament of the atlas, the apical and alar ligaments of the axis and the membrana tectoria (Figs 3.23–3.26). The **transverse ligament of the atlas** is a strong band which passes transversely across the posterior surface of the dens and attaches to paired tubercles on the medial aspect of the lateral masses of the atlas. This ligament serves to hold the dens in close proximity to the anterior arch of the atlas whilst permitting rotational movements at the joint. A thinner fibrous band passes upwards from the transverse ligament to attach to the basi-occiput, whilst

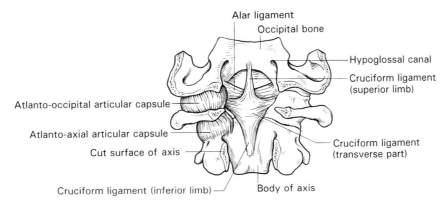

Fig. 3.23
The cruciform ligament of the axis.

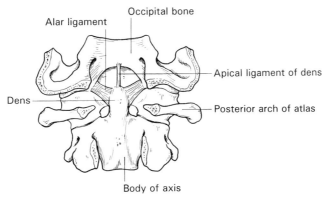

Fig. 3.24
Alar and apical ligaments of the axis.

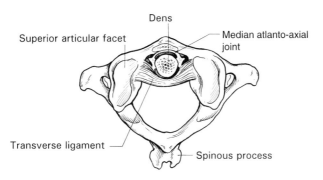

Fig. 3.25
Superior view of the median atlanto-axial joint.

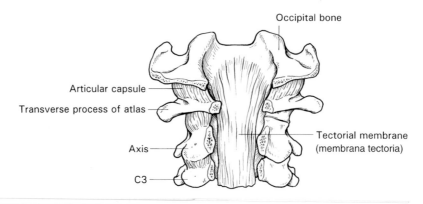

Fig. 3.26
Dorsal view of the membrana tectoria (tectorial membrane)

a second band passes downwards to attach to the posterior surface of the body of the axis. The combination of these two vertical bands together with the transverse ligament forms the **cruciform ligament** of the axis. The dens is attached to the occipital bone via the apical and alar ligaments. The **apical ligament** passes from the apex of the dens to the anterior margin of the foramen magnum, passing between the two alar ligaments and blending with the anterior atlanto-occipital membrane and the upper band of the cruciform ligament. The **alar ligaments** are strong, rounded cords which attach to the medial sides of the occipital condyles, passing from the flattened lateral facets on the dens. These ligaments are taut in flexion and relaxed in extension. The **membrana tectoria** is a

prolongation of the posterior longitudinal ligament which passes within the vertebral canal covering the dens and its ligaments. It passes from the posterior surface of the body of the axis superiorly to attach to the basi-occiput where it blends with the dura mater. The principal movement at the atlanto-axial junction is rotational (turning of the head on the neck), which is limited by tension in the opposing alar ligaments.

The **intervertebral joints** occur between both adjacent vertebral bodies and adjacent neural arches (Figs 3.27–3.31). The principal connection between the vertebral bodies are the **intervertebral discs** which occur between all vertebrae from the axis to the sacrum. They are generally thickest in the lumbar region and thinnest in the upper thoracic segment of

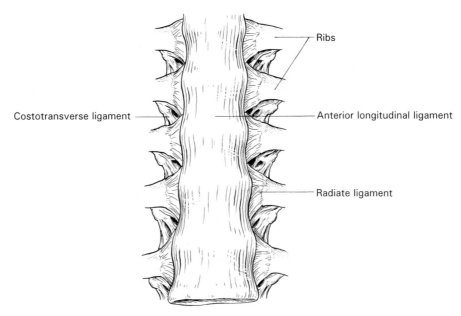

Fig. 3.27
Anterior longitudinal ligament.

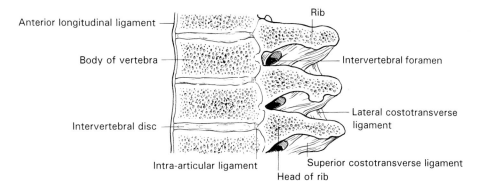

Fig. 3.28
Costotransverse articulations.

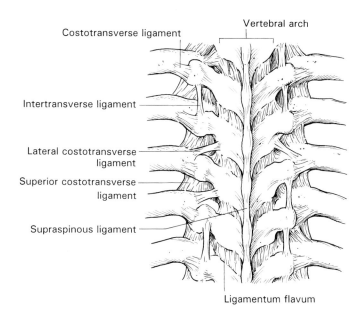

Fig. 3.29
Posterior view of the costovertebral joints.

the column. They adhere to the hyaline cartilage layers that cover both the inferior surface of the vertebral body above and that of the vertebral body below. Only the periphery of the disc has an arterial supply, with the greater part of the disc being avascular. The discs are also connected to the anterior longitudinal ligament in front and the posterior longitudinal ligament behind. They consist of an outer section of concentric fibrocartilaginous strands – the **annulus fibrosus** – and a central **nucleus pulposus**, which is the embryological remnant of the notochord. The **anterior longitudinal ligament** is a strong band which passes along the length of the vertebral column, being attached to the basi-occiput and anterior tubercle of the atlas above and to the front of the sacrum below. Along its length it is attached to the intervertebral discs but it is loose as it passes across the anterior surface of the vertebral

bodies. The **posterior longitudinal ligament** runs inside the vertebral canal and is attached to the posterior border of the body of the axis above and to the sacrum below. It therefore runs virtually the entire length of the column supporting the posterior aspect of the vertebral bodies and, like the anterior longitudinal ligament, it is firmly adherent to the intervertebral discs. It is continuous above with the membrana tectoria.

The neural arch components of the vertebral column overlap at the laminae and spinous processes and are connected by a series of ligaments, including the ligamenta flava, supraspinous ligaments, ligamentum nuchae, interspinous ligaments and intertransverse ligaments. The **ligamentum flavum** connects the laminae of adjacent vertebrae and extends from the region of the articular capsules of the intervertebral

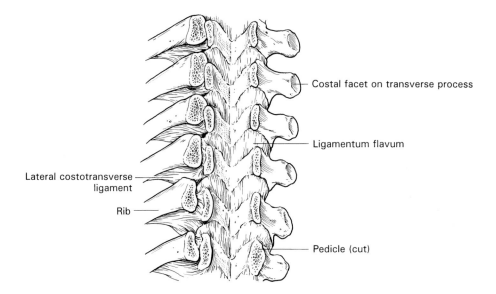

Fig. 3.30
Ligamentum flavum.

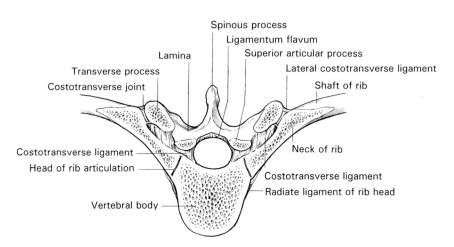

Fig. 3.31
Costovertebral joints.

joints to cover the area of the spine. It consists of a tough, yellow, elastic tissue which is thickest and displays the greatest degree of recoil in the lumbar region. Whilst this ligament permits the separation of the laminae during flexion of the trunk, it also acts to check and control the action. The **supraspinous ligaments** are strong, fibrous connections between the apices of the spinous processes. They extend from C7 to the sacrum and are thickest in the lumbar region. The **ligamentum nuchae** is homologous with the supraspinous ligaments and extends from the external occipital protuberance and occipital crest above, to the spinous process of C7. The **interspinous ligaments** are thick, almost membranous connections between adjacent spinous processes and each passes from the

root of a spinous process to its apex, so that it meets the ligamentum flavum in front and the supraspinous ligament behind. They are poorly defined in the cervical region and thickest in the lumbar segment of the column. Finally, the **intertransverse ligaments** pass between adjacent transverse processes. They are irregular in form in the cervical and lumbar regions but are well-defined rounded cords in the thoracic region.

Movements of the column as a whole are a combination of flexion, extension, lateral flexion and rotation. In **flexion** of the column the anterior longitudinal ligament is relaxed, the anterior region of the intervertebral discs is compressed and, at the limit of the movement, the posterior longitudinal ligament, interspinous and supraspinous ligaments and the posterior region of the intervertebral discs are taut. In **extension** the opposite situation arises, with the movement being limited by the contact of spinous processes and by tension in the anterior longitudinal ligament. **Lateral flexion** involves contraction of the musculature on one side of the trunk with concomitant relaxation on the opposite side. Compression of the intervertebral disc obviously occurs on the side that is in active flexion. **Rotation** involves a twisting action of the trunk with one vertebra rotating in relation to its neighbour which causes a twisting deformation in the intervertebral discs.

MENINGES

The central nervous system (brain and spinal cord) is surrounded by 3 continuous membranes or meninges which offer support and protection to the neural tissue (Fig. 3.32). The outermost, and strongest, layer is the **dura mater** which is separated from the inner **arachnoid mater** by the **subdural space**. The **subarachnoid space** separates the arachnoid mater from the deepest **pia mater**, which is firmly bound to the underlying neural tissue. The arrangement of the meninges is sufficiently different in the intracranial and spinal regions to merit separate descriptions.

Intracranial meninges and dural venous sinuses
The **dura mater** is a tough, fibrous, bilaminar sheet with an outer (endosteal) layer which lines the bones of

the intracranial cavity and is continuous with the pericranium through the foramina and sutures. This layer has a rich arterial supply from the anterior, middle and posterior meningeal arteries. The supratentorial dural nerve supply is from the ophthalmic division of the trigeminal cranial nerve, whilst the infratentorial region is supplied via the vagus and the upper 3 cervical spinal nerves. The inner (meningeal) layer is generally firmly bound to the endosteal layer but separates from it in specific locations, forming a cavity for the dural venous sinuses. In other specific locations, the meningeal layer of dura becomes stretched and forms folds which occur as septa to separate specific regions of the brain. There are 2 principal septa (falx cerebri and tentorium cerebelli), which serve to subdivide the cranial cavity into compartments that support the brain and prevent excessive movement within the cranial cavity (Figs 3.33 and 3.34) The **falx cerebri** is a vertical fold of meningeal dura which separates the two cerebral hemispheres. It extends from the crista galli of the ethmoid bone anteriorly to the horizontal tentorium cerebelli and internal occipital protuberance posteriorly. The superior sagittal sinus runs in its fixed upper border, whilst the inferior sagittal sinus runs in its free lower border. The **tentorium cerebelli** is a horizontal fold of meningeal dura which separates the occipital lobes above from the cerebellar hemispheres below. It has a fixed and a free border. The fixed border is attached anteriorly to the posterior clinoid processes of the dorsum sella, laterally to the superior edges of

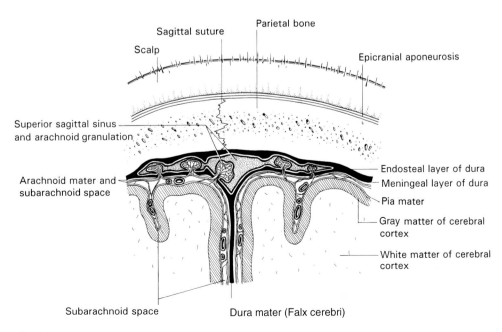

Fig. 3.32
The meninges at the sagittal suture.

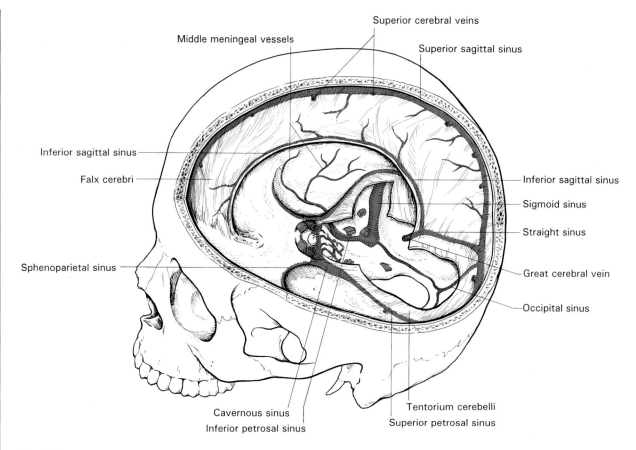

Fig. 3.33
The dural venous sinuses.

the petrous temporal bone, and posteriorly to the occipital grooves on the squamous part of the occipital bone. The free border is attached anteriorly to the anterior clinoid processes and forms the tentorial notch through which the midbrain passes. The superior petrosal sinuses run in the petrosal region of the fixed border of the tentorium and the transverse sinuses run in the occipital attachments. The straight sinus is formed at the junction between the falx cerebri and the tentorium cerebelli by the union of the inferior sagittal sinus with the great cerebral vein.

The dural venous sinuses are valveless spaces, sited between the two layers of dura mater, and the majority ultimately drain into the internal jugular veins. The **superior sagittal sinus** runs in the upper border of the falx cerebri and extends from the foramen caecum in front to the internal occipital protuberance behind. Here, it generally becomes continuous with the **right transverse sinus** which runs in the fixed border of the tentorium cerebelli. The **inferior sagittal sinus** runs in the lower free border of the falx cerebri and is joined by the **great cerebral vein** to form the **straight sinus** at the junction between the vertical falx cerebri and the horizontal tentorium cerebelli. The straight sinus passes posteriorly and generally becomes continuous

with the **left transverse sinus** at the confluence of the sinuses. The paired transverse sinuses become the **sigmoid sinuses** as they pass inferiorly in the mastoid region and then exit through the jugular foramen to become the **internal jugular veins** when they are joined by the inferior petrosal sinus. Each transverse sinus also receives the **superior petrosal sinus**, which runs laterally along the petrous temporal ridge from the cavernous sinus. The **inferior petrosal sinus** also passes from the cavernous sinus but passes lateral to the clivus and exits through the jugular foramen before joining with the sigmoid sinus to form the internal jugular vein. A small **occipital sinus** runs in the falx cerebelli, which is a small vertical fold of meningeal dura that separates the cerebellar hemispheres. The **cavernous sinuses** are situated lateral to the body of the sphenoid bone in the middle cranial fossa. Each is traversed by an internal carotid artery, its sympathetic plexus and the abducens nerve. In the lateral wall of each sinus run the oculomotor and trochlear nerves along with the ophthalmic and maxillary divisions of the trigeminal nerve. The cavernous sinuses connect anteriorly with the ophthalmic veins and each receives a **sphenoparietal sinus** which runs medially along the lesser wing of the sphenoid bone. Posteriorly, the

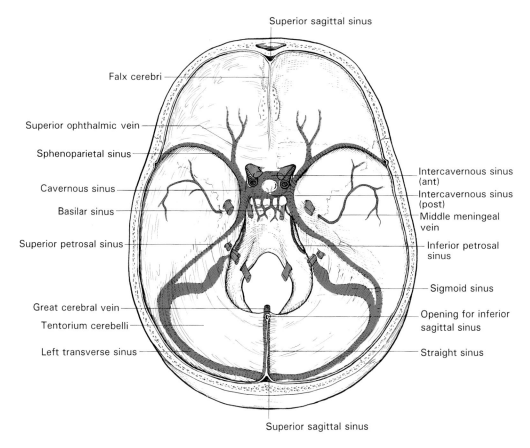

Superior sagittal sinus

Falx cerebri

Superior ophthalmic vein

Sphenoparietal sinus

Cavernous sinus

Basilar sinus

Superior petrosal sinus

Great cerebral vein

Tentorium cerebelli

Left transverse sinus

Intercavernous sinus (ant)

Intercavernous sinus (post)

Middle meningeal vein

Inferior petrosal sinus

Sigmoid sinus

Opening for inferior sagittal sinus

Straight sinus

Superior sagittal sinus

Fig. 3.34
The cranial base and the dural venous sinuses.

cavernous sinuses drain via the superior and inferior petrosal sinuses. A number of emissary veins connect the cavernous sinuses to deeper venous plexuses, e.g. the pterygoid plexus, pharyngeal plexus etc. Further, the paired cavernous sinuses are interconnected via channels in the diaphragma sella.

The **subdural** space lies between the dura mater and the arachnoid mater and is traversed by cerebral veins en route to the superior sagittal sinus. The **arachnoid mater** is a delicate and a vascular membrane which bridges the sulci of the brain and lies sandwiched between the more superficial dura mater and the deeper pia mater. The region between the arachnoid mater and the pia mater is the important **subarachnoid space**. This contains the cerebrospinal fluid that bathes the brain as well as the cerebral arteries and veins. The width of the space varies, so that it is narrow over the gyri of the brain but deeper in the region of the sulci. The space is widest at the base of the brain, where a number of named subarachnoid cisterns occur, and so cerebrospinal fluid accumulates in these locations. The subarachnoid space extends into the superior sagittal sinus via arachnoid granulations. These granulations allow cerebrospinal fluid to drain from the subarachnoid space into the dural venous system.

The **pia mater** is the deepest layer of the meninges. It is an impermeable vascular membrane which follows closely the contours of the brain surface and is not easily separated from the neural tissue that it covers.

Spinal meninges

The **spinal dura** is a single-layered structure representing only the equivalent of the meningeal dura of the intracranial region, whereas the equivalent of the endosteal layer is the periosteum which covers the bony surfaces of the vertebral canal. The **extradural** (epidural) space is the area between the spinal dura and the periosteum (Fig. 3.35) and it is filled with areolar tissue and valveless venous plexuses.

At the foramen magnum, the periosteum and spinal dura fuse and indeed in the upper cervical region they may come into close enough contact to virtually eliminate any extradural space. Thus, a solution injected into the extradural space cannot extend further cranially than the foramen magnum or, in some instances, the upper cervical levels.

The spinal dura is firmly attached to the margins of the foramen magnum and the posterior surfaces of the

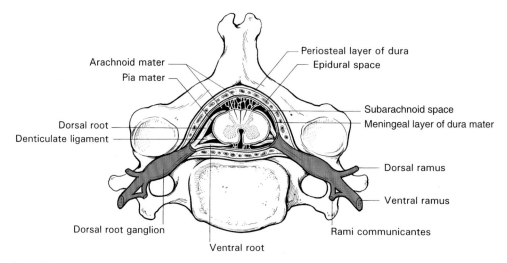

Fig. 3.35
Transverse section at the level of C4.

bodies of the first and second cervical vertebrae and small fibrous slips connect the dura anteriorly to the posterior longitudinal ligament. Therefore, the spinal dura is only free and loose on its posterior aspect. The dural sac (containing the spinal cord, nerve roots, blood vessels and cerebrospinal fluid) extends inferiorly to approximately the level of S2 in the adult, where it is pierced by the filum terminale (a continuation of the pia mater). It attaches to the periosteum on the posterior surface of the coccyx and is covered by spinal dura. One of its functions is to stabilize both the dural sac and the spinal cord.

The outer boundary of the extradural space is formed by the periosteum, whilst the dural sac forms the inner boundary and tends to occupy a more anterior position in the vertebral canal. This serves to separate the space into a small anterior and two larger posterolateral components. The distance from the posterior border of the space to the dural sac varies from 1 mm in the cervical region to approximately 6 mm in the lumbar region. Dorsal midline strands connect the spinal dura to the ligamentum flavum and these cause a fold in the dura – the **plica mediana dorsalis**, which narrows the extradural space in the midline (Fig. 3.36). Connective tissue bands have also been demonstrated extending laterally from the plica mediana dorsalis, thus subdividing the posterolateral compartments into anterior and posterior sections. The posterior longitudinal ligament which runs down the posterior aspect of the vertebral bodies and discs has numerous connections to the anterior region of the dural sac. The close proximity of the dural sac to the anterior wall of the vertebral canal can isolate the ventral compartment and so prevent entry of fluid from the dorsal parts of the extradural space.

The extradural space extends around the spinal nerves for a short distance as they exit through the intervertebral foramen. These exit sites tend to increase in diameter from above downwards, especially between C5–T1 and L4–S1 through which the large spinal nerves pass for the innervation of the limbs. The dorsal and ventral roots of a spinal nerve cross the extradural space from the dural sac to the intervertebral foramen. The nerves lie in the posterolateral aspect of the space and become progressively longer and more oblique in orientation as the cord is descended. At the intervertebral foramen, the nerve (together with fat and blood vessels) is tethered to the walls by connective tissue strands known as Sharpey's ligaments. With increasing age, the foramina present an increasing barrier (sometimes to the point of complete occlusion) to the successful and uninterrupted communication between the vertebral canal and the rest of the body.

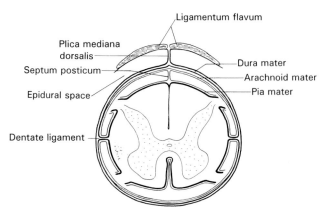

Fig. 3.36
Transverse section to show the spinal meninges.

Extradural fat is highly vascular, with a semi-fluid consistency, and fills much of the remainder of the extradural space. The amount of fat is not proportional to total body fat and tends to vary with age, offering increasing resistance to injection. The **extradural veins** (plexus of Batson) are large and valveless and lie mainly in the anterolateral region of the extradural space. They have numerous connections at all segmental levels including the sacral (and therefore iliac and uterine) venous plexus and the abdominal and thoracic veins. The pressure changes within the body cavities are reflected in the extradural veins and this is particularly relevant during pregnancy, when the veins become distended, effectively decreasing the volume of the extradural space.

The **subdural space** is a potential space that exists between the spinal layer of dura and the arachnoid mater. It extends as far inferiorly as the subdural cistern at the level of S2 and is continuous for a short distance around the exiting spinal nerves.

The **spinal arachnoid mater** is a thin, delicate membrane which loosely covers the spinal cord. It is continuous above with the cerebral arachnoid mater and widens out below where it invests the cauda equina. It terminates at the level of S2.

The **spinal subarachnoid space** is relatively wide in the spinal region and is continuous above with the cerebral space. It terminates at the S2 level and is partially divided by 2 septa – the subarachnoid septum and the ligamentum denticulum of the pia mater (Fig. 3.37). Several connective tissue strands or trabeculae are found in this space, and although their pattern varies considerably between individuals, they do tend to be more numerous along the dorsal aspect of the cord. In most individuals, a midline dorsal septum (septum posticum) extends from the mid-cervical to the lumbar regions. This septum usually has irregular perforations and tends to be increasingly fenestrated towards its upper and lower ends. It is generally attached to the pia mater along the course of the spinal cord and tends to thicken with increasing age.

Lateral to the septum posticum, 2 dorsolateral septae extend from the region of the dorsal rootlets, which they attach to the dorsal arachnoid mater. The dorsolateral septae tend to be more irregular and fenestrated than the septum posticum and generally extend further rostrally and caudally, probably serving to tether the dorsal rootlets and keep them clear of the lateral parts of the spinal cord. Unlike the septum posticum, these trabeculations tend to atrophy with age. More substantial lateral projections from the pia, known as the denticulate ligaments, attach to the dura mater and act to support the spinal cord. There are no further attachments of the pia anterior to the denticulate ligaments.

The **spinal pia mater** is thicker and less vascular than its cerebral counterpart. It is firmly bound to the spinal cord and forms an intimate sheath around the

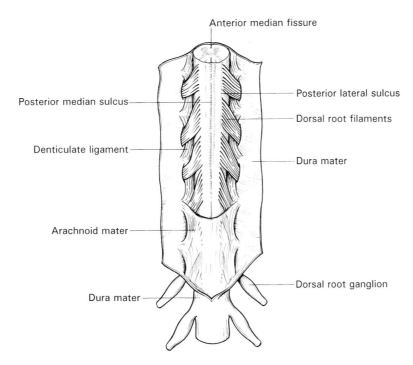

Fig. 3.37
Dorsal view of the spinal cord and meninges.

spinal nerves. It is continuous above with the cerebral dura and terminates below as the filum terminale, which attaches to the dorsum of the coccyx. The pia is thickened in the midline to form the **linea splendens**, which fills the anterior median sulcus of the spinal cord. In addition, the lateral aspects of the pia are elongated to form the ligamentum denticulatum (Fig. 3.37). This lateral area of the pia forms a series of 21 tooth-like projections which cross the subarachnoid space to fuse with the arachnoid mater. The first tooth arises posterior to the level of the vertebral artery, where it pierces the dura mater, and the last tooth arises between the exit points of the last thoracic and first lumbar spinal nerves. The posterior region of the pia over the posterior median septum is also raised and projects into the subarachnoid space as the subarachnoid septum.

CEREBROSPINAL FLUID

Cerebrospinal fluid (CSF) is formed via choroid plexuses in the ventricles of the brain. Where the pia mater and its blood vessels come into contact with the ependymal lining of the ventricles, a double membrane (tela choroidea) is formed. This is the vascularized membrane of the choroid plexus and produces the CSF. As they are the largest, most of the CSF is produced in the **lateral ventricles** from where it passes to the **third ventricle** via the paired **interventricular foramina**. A small amount of CSF is produced in the third ventricle, which is connected to the **fourth ventricle** (anterior to the cerebellum) via the **cerebral aqueduct**. Further production of CSF occurs in the fourth ventricle as a choroid plexus is present in its roof and from here the CSF eventually escapes into the subarachnoid space via 3 foramina or defects in the roof of the fourth ventricle: the median **foramen of Magendie** and two lateral **foramina of Luschka**. Below the level of the fourth ventricle, a central canal extends downwards as a tiny tube throughout the length of the spinal cord and into the upper end of the filum terminale. Re-absorption of the CSF into the vascular system occurs via the **arachnoid granulations** into the superior sagittal venous sinus.

CSF is a clear fluid and its function is to support and protect the brain and spinal cord. The total volume in the adult is approximately 130 ml and the average daily production is 150 ml. Spinal CSF accounts only for some 35 ml of the total and although some may drain into local venous plexuses, most returns to the cranium for disposal. A combination of diffusion and alterations in posture results in the slow circulation of CSF.

CSF COMPOSITION

H⁺	32–36 nmol/L
Glucose	1.5–4.0 nmol/L
Sodium	140–150 mmol/L
Chloride	120–130 mmol/L
Bicarbonate	25–30 mmol/L
Protein	0.15–0.3 g/L
Osmolality	280 mOsm at 37°C
Normal pressure in lumbar region	60–100 mmHg in lateral position 200–250 mmHg in sitting position

BRAIN

Topographically, the brain can be separated into the forebrain, midbrain and hindbrain (Fig. 3.38). The forebrain is further divided into the telencephalon and diencephalon. The **telencephalon** consists of paired cerebral hemispheres which are partially separated by a deep longitudinal fissure containing the falx cerebri. The cortex of each hemisphere is marked by a series of ridges (gyri) and troughs (sulci) and is separated into lobes (Fig. 3.39). The **frontal lobes** lie anterior to the central sulcus and occupy the anterior cranial fossa. The **parietal lobes** run backwards from the central sulcus, above the lateral fissure, to the parieto-occipital sulcus. The **occipital lobes** lie between the parieto-occipital sulcus and the pre-occipital notch, filling the region of the posterior cranial fossa above the tentorium cerebelli. The **temporal lobes** lie in the middle cranial fossa and are bounded above by the lateral fissure.

The **diencephalon** lies between the cerebral hemispheres and the midbrain and is the location of the thalamus, hypothalamus and epithalamus. At the free border of the tentorium cerebelli, the midbrain connects the forebrain to the hindbrain. The **hindbrain** consists of the pons, medulla oblongata and cerebellum. The **pons** is located at the level of the clivus, which is the median slope of bone in the posterior cranial fossa formed from the fusion of the sphenoid and occipital bones. The **medulla oblongata** passes out through the foramen magnum to become continuous with the spinal cord. The cerebellar hemispheres sit in the posterior cranial fossa below the level of the tentorium cerebelli.

The brain derives its blood supply from both the paired internal carotid arteries and the vertebral

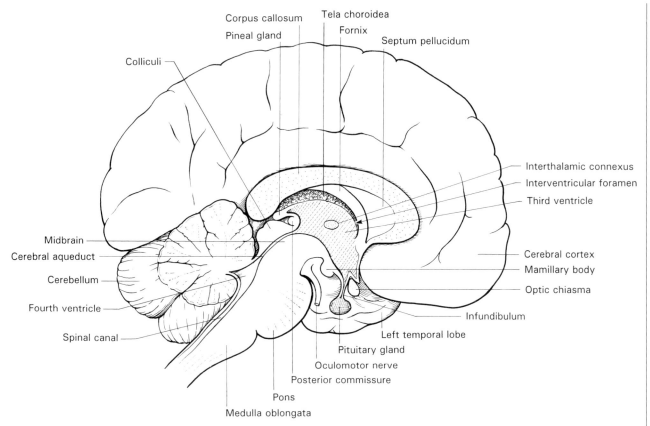

Fig. 3.38
Sagittal section through the brain and brainstem.

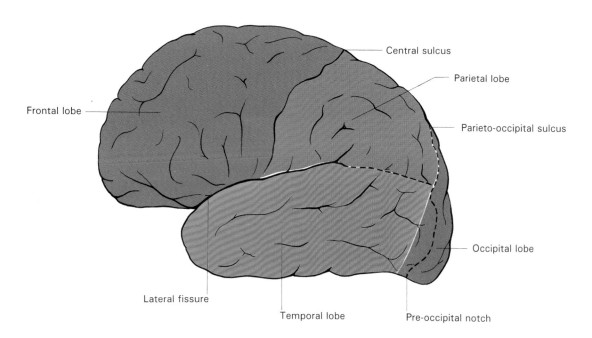

Fig. 3.39
The left cerebral hemisphere.

arteries (Fig. 3.40). These unite to form a circle on the base of the brain from which the anterior, middle and posterior cerebral arteries arise (Fig. 3.41). The venous drainage of the brain tissue is largely via the dural venous sinuses, which ultimately drain into the internal jugular veins.

CRANIAL NERVES

Examination of the base of the brain shows the location of the 12 pairs of cranial nerves (Fig. 3.42). The olfactory tract (I) can be found on the inferior surface of the frontal lobe and the optic nerve (II) lies anterior to the pituitary stalk in the interpeduncular fossa. The oculomotor nerve (III) appears at the junction between the midbrain and the pons and the trochlear nerve (IV) winds around from the posterior surface of the

midbrain to exit from the brain lateral to the oculomotor nerve. The trigeminal nerve (V) exits from the ventral surface of the pons, whilst the abducens nerve (VI) exits at the pontomedullary junction in the midline. The facial (VII) and vestibulocochlear (VIII) nerves also exit at the pontomedullary junction but are more laterally placed. The glossopharyngeal (IX), vagus (X) and cranial part of the accessory (XI) nerves exit from the medulla oblongata, lateral to the olive, by a series of rootlets. The spinal part of the accessory nerve exits from the upper segments of the spinal cord, ascends through the foramen magnum, joins with the cranial part, and together they exit through the jugular foramen before separating again into spinal and cranial components. The hypoglossal nerve (XII) exits from the medulla oblongata lateral to the pyramids by a series of rootlets.

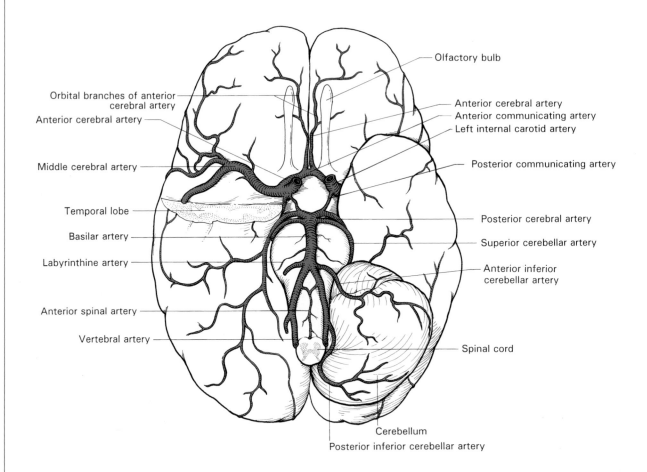

Fig. 3.40
The arteries of the brain.

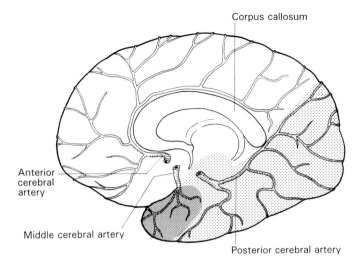

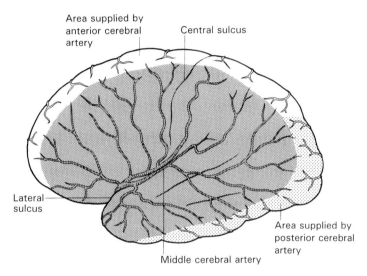

Fig. 3.41
The cortical distribution of the cerebral arteries.

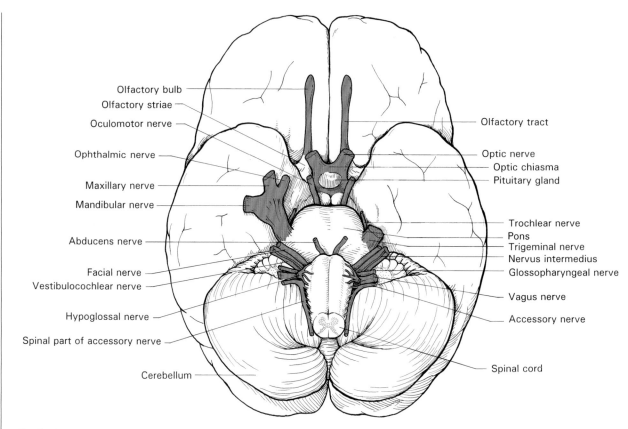

Fig. 3.42
The cranial nerves at the base of the brain.

Cranial nerve I – the olfactory nerve (Fig. 3.43)

The olfactory epithelium lies in the roof of the nose and occupies only some 2 cm² of space. The olfactory nerves are bipolar neurons that pass from the ciliated receptor in the olfactory epithelium, converge and pass through the cribriform plate of the ethmoid bone to terminate in the olfactory bulb (Fig. 3.42). Secondary neurons then pass along the olfactory tract, adjacent to the inferior surface of the frontal lobe, before bifurcating into medial and lateral olfactory striae at the anterior perforated substance. The lateral striae terminate in the primary olfactory cortex of the uncus whilst the medial olfactory striae project to the septal area of the cortex. Fractures affecting the anterior cranial fossa can result in a tearing of the olfactory nerves leading to anosmia, an inability to perceive smell. A loss of smell is also associated with a reduced sensation of taste.

Cranial nerve II – the optic nerve (Figs 3.44 and 3.45)

Both the optic nerve and the retina develop directly from an outgrowth of the forebrain vesicle and as such the optic nerve is better described as a tract rather than a nerve. The retina is essentially a four-layer membrane

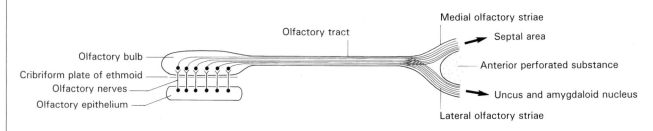

Fig. 3.43
The olfactory nerve.

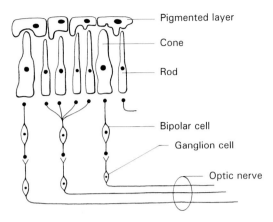

Fig. 3.44
The retina.

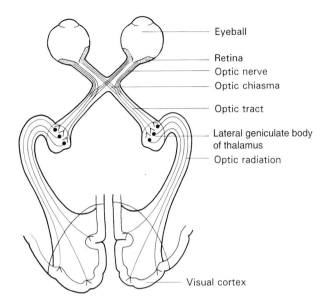

Fig. 3.45
The optic pathway.

(Fig. 3.44). The outermost layer houses the pigment cells that react to light stimulus and set up the electrical impulses that are conveyed to the second layer of receptor cells (rods and cones). The rods are more numerous and whereas they are more sensitive in conditions of low illumination, the cones are more sensitive to colour and detail. Neural transmission from the photoreceptor cells to the bipolar cells of the third layer is convergent for the rods and essentially non-convergent for the more discriminative cones. The bipolar cells then synapse on the fourth layer of ganglion cells, whose axons form the optic nerve.

Each optic nerve passes backwards from the eye, through the optic canal in company with the ophthalmic artery, to the optic chiasma in the interpeduncular fossa anterior to the hypophyseal infundibulum (Fig. 3.42). At the chiasma, fibers from the nasal half of the retina cross to the opposite side and unite with fibers from the ipsilateral temporal retinal projection before becoming the optic tract (Fig. 3.45). Each optic tract then extends from the chiasma around the midbrain to terminate in the lateral geniculate body of the thalamus. Some fibers will leave in the superior brachium to terminate in the superior colliculus, thereby subserving reflex movements. The final neuron pathway connects the thalamus to the primary visual cortex via the optic radiation (geniculocalcarine tract). The primary visual cortex centres around the calcarine sulcus of the occipital lobe (Figs 3.39 and 3.45).

Defects in the visual pathway are usually described in terms of loss of fields of vision. The pathway is vulnerable to damage in a number of locations, e.g. the nerve, the chiasma, the tract etc. Damage can arise from trauma, aneurysms (usually of the internal carotid artery), tumors (often pituitary), thrombosis, etc.

Cranial nerve III – the oculomotor nerve (Figs 3.46 and 3.47)

The oculomotor nerve carries somatic efferent fibers for the innervation of all the extra-ocular muscles except the superior oblique and the lateral rectus. The upper motor neurons originate in the precentral cortex and travel down through the posterior limb of the internal capsule before synapsing in the oculomotor nucleus in the peri-aqueductal gray matter at the superior collicular level of the midbrain (Fig. 3.7). From the nucleus, the lower motor neurons pass forward and exit from the brain in the interpeduncular fossa (Fig. 3.42). The nerve then passes forwards into the lateral wall of the cavernous sinus and traverses the superior orbital fissure to gain access to the orbit. It then splits into superior and inferior divisions, with the former supplying the superior rectus and levator palpebrae superioris and the latter supplying the inferior oblique and the medial and inferior recti.

The oculomotor nerve also carries a parasympathetic efferent component which supplies the sphincter pupillae and the ciliary muscle. These fibers originate in the accessory oculomotor nucleus (Edinger–Westphal) of the midbrain and pass to the ciliary ganglion within the orbit, via the branch of the oculomotor nerve that supplies the inferior oblique muscle. The postganglionic fibers then leave the ganglion as short ciliary nerves to supply the sphincter

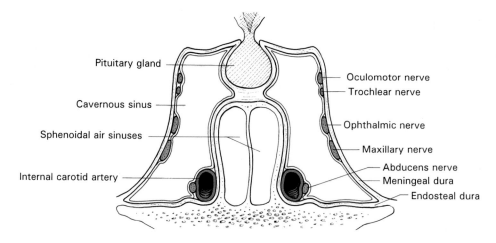

Fig. 3.46
Relationship of the cranial nerves to the cavernous sinuses.

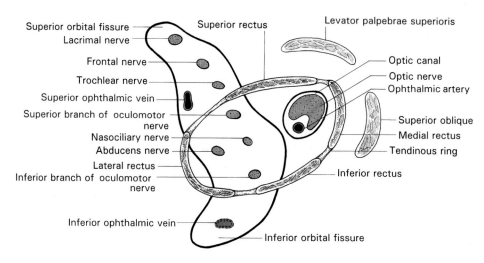

Fig. 3.47
The right superior orbital fissure and optic canal.

pupillae and the ciliary muscle. Some postganglionic sympathetic fibers from the internal carotid plexus also pass via this route to supply structures within the orbit.

Damage to the oculomotor nerve can occur following a subdural hematoma or tumor above the tentorium cerebelli, forcing the cerebral peduncles inferiorly into the tentorial incisure. Aneurysms of the posterior cerebral and posterior communicating arteries can also cause pressure on the nerve.

During clinical testing for the integrity of the oculomotor nerve, each muscle is examined in its position of greatest efficiency. The patient is asked to look:

1. upwards and laterally to test the superior rectus
2. downwards and laterally to test the inferior rectus
3. upwards and medially to test the inferior oblique
4. medially to test the medial rectus.

A complete section of the third cranial nerve will result in:

1. ptosis because of paralysis to the levator palpebrae superioris
2. lateral strabismus due to the unopposed action of the lateral rectus and superior oblique muscles
3. dilation of the pupil due to paralysis of the sphincter pupillae muscle
4. loss of accommodation of the light reflex due to paralysis of the sphincter pupillae and the ciliary muscle
5. proptosis owing to relaxation of the ocular muscles
6. diplopia.

Cranial nerve IV – the trochlear nerve (Figs 3.46 and 3.47)

This is the most slender of all the cranial nerves and supplies just one striated intra-ocular muscle – the superior oblique. The nerve derives its name from the fact that the tendon of the superior oblique muscle passes through a cartilaginous 'pulley-like' sling on the way to its insertion into the sclera of the eyeball. The trochlear motor nucleus is located in the periaqueductal gray matter of the midbrain at the level of the inferior colliculus (Fig. 3.7). The lower motor neurons decussate dorsal to the cerebral aqueduct before emerging from the dorsal surface of the brainstem. The nerve then winds around the cerebral peduncles to the ventral surface of the brainstem (Fig. 3.42) and passes into the lateral wall of the cavernous sinus lying inferior to the oculomotor nerve and superior to the ophthalmic division of the trigeminal nerve. It enters the orbit through the superior orbital fissure and passes superior to the common tendinous ring to reach the superior oblique muscle.

The trochlear nerve is rarely damaged, but pressure can arise from aneurysms in the posterior cerebral artery. Damage to the trochlear nerve will result in diplopia and an inability to look downwards and laterally with the affected eye.

Cranial nerve V – the trigeminal nerve (Figs 3.48–3.50)

This is the largest of the cranial nerves and carries both motor and sensory information. It has 3 divisions – ophthalmic, maxillary and mandibular, which exit from the ventral surface of the pons (Fig. 3.42).

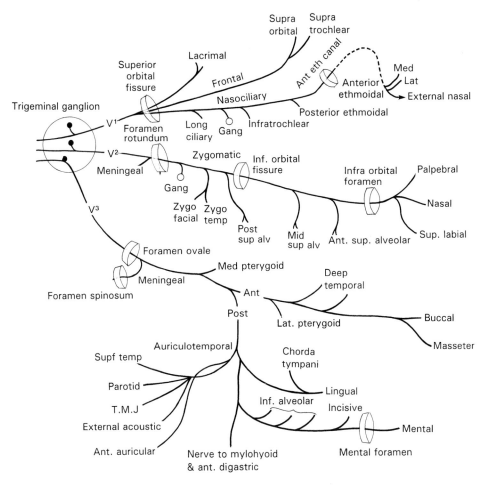

Fig. 3.48
Peripheral distribution of the trigeminal nerve.

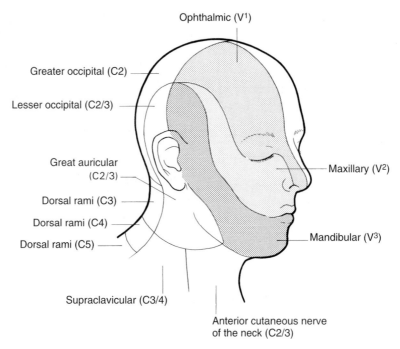

Fig. 3.49
Cutaneous distribution of the trigeminal nerve.

The ophthalmic nerve

This is the smallest of the divisions and is purely sensory in nature supplying the superior part of the face and anterior part of the scalp (Fig. 3.49). The ophthalmic nerve has 3 branches, which arise before the nerve enters the orbit through the superior orbital fissure (Fig. 3.48):

1. the **frontal nerve** bifurcates into a large supra-orbital nerve which supplies the skin of the upper eyelid and scalp and a smaller supratrochlear nerve which supplies the skin of the forehead
2. the **nasociliary nerve** gives off several branches:
   a. long ciliary nerves to the eyeball
   b. ganglionic branches to the ciliary ganglion
   c. posterior and anterior ethmoidal nerves to the ethmoidal air sinuses and nasal cavity, and
   d. the infratrochlear nerve, which supplies the medial aspect of the upper eyelid and the lacrimal sac.
3. the **lacrimal nerve** supplies the lacrimal gland and the adjoining conjunctiva before ending in the skin of the upper eyelid.

The maxillary nerve

This is also a purely sensory nerve, supplying the region of the face below the corner of the eyelid and above the corner of the mouth (Fig. 3.49). The nerve leaves the intracranial region through the foramen rotundum to enter the pterygopalatine fossa. It passes laterally through the pterygomaxillary fissure to enter the infratemporal fossa and then travels through the inferior orbital fissure, where it continues as the infra-orbital nerve, exiting from the infra-orbital foramen on the face.

The maxillary division has several branches:

1. **Meningeal branches** arise from the main trunk while it is still within the cranium and supply the dura matter
2. **ganglionic branches** arise within the pterygopalatine fossa and enter the pterygopalatine ganglion.
3. The **zygomatic nerve** also arises in the pterygopalatine fossa and divides into the zygomaticofacial and the zygomaticotemporal nerves. The former is distributed to the skin of the temple and the latter to the skin over the prominence of the cheek
4. The **posterior superior alveolar nerve** arises in pterygopalatine fossa and descends under the mucous lining of the maxillary sinus. It supplies the sinus and, via a plexus, goes on to supply the maxillary molar teeth, associated gums and the adjoining part of the cheek.
5. The **middle superior alveolar nerve** arises from the infra-orbital nerve and runs downwards into the maxillary sinus. Like the posterior superior alveolar nerve it supplies the sinus and, via a dental plexus, supplies the upper premolar teeth.

6. the **anterior superior alveolar nerve** also arises from the infra-orbital nerve and passes downwards into the maxillary sinus. It supplies the sinus and, via a dental plexus, supplies the incisor and canine teeth. In addition, it gives off a small nasal branch that supplies the mucous membrane of the anterior part of the lateral wall of the nose.
7. once the infra-orbital nerve has exited through the infra-orbital foramen it terminates in 3 groups:
   a. **palpebral branches** to the lateral angle of the eye and the lower eyelid
   b. **nasal branches** to the skin of the side of the nose
   c. **superior labial branches** to the skin of the anterior part of the cheek, the upper lip and the mucous membrane of the mouth and labial glands.

The mandibular nerve

This is a mixed nerve carrying both motor and sensory components. The mandibular division exits through the foramen ovale in the skull, giving off 2 branches, one sensory and one motor, before it bifurcates into a small anterior and a larger posterior trunk. The sensory meningeal branch re-enters the skull through the foramen spinosum to supply the dura mater of the middle cranial fossa. The motor branch is the nerve to the medial pterygoid muscle, which also goes on to supply the tensor tympani and the tensor veli palatini muscles (Fig. 3.48).

Anterior trunk:

1. The **buccal nerve** supplies the skin over the anterior part of the buccinator muscle and the mucous membrane of the buccal surface of the lower gum.
2. The **masseteric nerve** is motor to the masseter muscle and also supplies a small filament to the temporomandibular joint.
3. The **deep temporal nerves**, usually two, supply the temporalis muscle.
4. The **nerve to the lateral pterygoid** muscle.

Posterior trunk:

1. The **auriculotemporal nerve** arises from 2 roots that surround the middle meningeal artery. It passes backwards and eventually terminates in 5 branches:
   a. the anterior auricular branch to the tragus and helix of the ear
   b. external acoustic branches to the skin of the meatus and tympanic membrane
   c. articular branches to the temporomandibular joint
   d. parotid branches conveying parasympathetic secretomotor fibers to the parotid gland
   e. superficial temporal branches to the skin of the temporal region.

2. The **lingual nerve** passes downwards and is joined by the chorda tympani branch of the facial nerve. It is sensory to the mucous membrane of the floor of the mouth, the lingual surface of the gums, and the mucous membrane of the presulcal part of the tongue.
3. the **inferior alveolar nerve** passes down towards the mandible and enters the mandibular foramen. It travels within the mandibular canal where it supplies the lower teeth and associated gums before terminating in incisive and mental branches. The former supplies the lower canine and incisor teeth and associated gums, whilst the latter passes out through the mental foramen and supplies the skin of the chin and the mucous membrane of the lower lip. Before the inferior alveolar nerve enters the mandibular foramen, it gives off the **nerve to mylohyoid** which supplies both the muscle of that name and the anterior belly of digastric.

Central connections of the trigeminal nerve (Fig. 3.50)

Sensory

The cell bodies of most of the sensory neurons in the trigeminal nerve are located in the trigeminal ganglion which sits in the cavum trigeminale on the anterior surface of the petrous temporal ridge. The 3 divisions of the trigeminal nerve converge on the ganglion before entering the CNS at the ventral surface of the pons. Primary neurons carrying discriminative touch information terminate in the principal sensory nucleus in the dorsal pons. Neurons carrying the sensory modalities of pain, temperature, light touch and pressure descend and terminate in the spinal nucleus of the trigeminal. This nucleus is continuous with the principal sensory nucleus above and extends down to the level of the second cervical spinal segment. The pars rostralis and interpolaris are associated with light touch and pressure sensations, whilst the pars caudalis is the ultimate destination of fibers carrying pain and temperature information. There is a somatotopic representation of the 3 divisions of the trigeminal nerve in the spinal nucleus: the mandibular fibers occupy a dorsal position, the maxillary fibers are more central and the ophthalmic fibers are located ventrally. Further, the ophthalmic input extends down to the cervical level whilst the maxillary input terminates rostral to this and the mandibular does not pass caudad to the mid-medullary level.

Proprioception

There is an acute awareness of intra-oral proprioception in particular, and neurons carrying proprioceptive information bypass the trigeminal

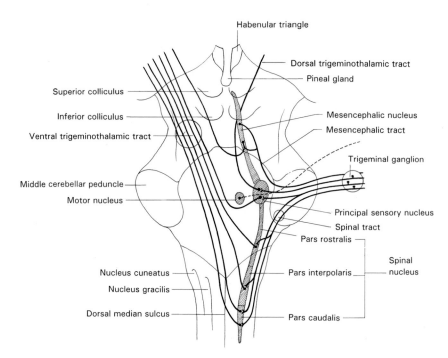

Fig. 3.50
Central connections of the trigeminal nerve.

ganglion to enter the CNS at the ventral pons and terminate in the mesencephalic nucleus. The majority of these fibres originate in the maxillary and mandibular divisions which is to be expected given the high level of intra-oral proprioception that is essential to both mastication and phonation. As well as receiving afferents from the masticatory muscles, the temporomandibular joint and periodontal ligaments of the teeth, there is also an input from proprioceptors in the extra-ocular and facial muscles. The mesencephalic nucleus is continuous with the principal sensory nucleus below and extends upwards into the dorsal pons and midbrain.

Central projections
The central projections of the trigeminal nerve are thalamic, cerebellar and nuclear. Thalamic projection fibers from the spinal nucleus decussate and ascend to the thalamus in the ventral trigeminothalamic tract. Most thalamic fibers from the principal sensory nucleus also decussate and ascend in the ventral trigeminothalamic tract but some remain ipsilateral and ascend in the uncrossed dorsal trigeminothalamic tract. Cerebellar projection fibers from the mesencephalic nucleus pass to the cerebellum via the superior cerebellar peduncles, whilst those from the spinal nucleus enter via the inferior cerebellar peduncles. Nuclear projection fibres pass to cranial nerves such as the facial and hypoglossal and do so by reflex arcs.

Motor
The trigeminal motor nucleus is located in the dorsal pons, medial to the principal sensory nucleus (Figs. 3.7 and 3.50). The lower motor neurons exit from the nucleus and pass out of the CNS at the ventral pons. The neurons then bypass the trigeminal ganglion and travel with the mandibular division of the trigeminal nerve, through the foramen ovale to supply the muscles of mastication (temporalis, masseter, pterygoids) as well as the tensor tympani, tensor veli palatini, mylohyoid and the anterior belly of digastric.

The trigeminal nerve is well protected as it lies so deep and is therefore seldom damaged apart from facial cuts which may sever minor cutaneous terminal branches. Lesions of the trigeminal nerve are not common but will result in sensory deprivation in the affected area. If this involves the mandibular division then there will also be motor loss to the muscles of mastication. Herpes zoster (shingles) has a predilection for the ophthalmic division and frequently leads to corneal ulceration.

Cranial nerve VI – the abducens nerve (Figs 3.46 and 3.47)

The abducens nerve carries only somatic efferent fibers to innervate the lateral rectus muscle of the eye. The motor nucleus is situated beneath the facial colliculus in the floor of the fourth ventricle (Fig. 3.7). Lower motor neurons exit from the nucleus, pass downwards and exit from the brainstem at the pontomedullary junction (Fig. 3.42). The nerve then passes forwards and pierces the dural lining of the posterior cranial fossa to enter the cavernous sinus where it lies lateral to the internal carotid artery. The nerve enters the orbit through the superior orbital fissure, passes through the tendinous ring for the rectus muscles, and runs forwards on the deep surface of the lateral rectus muscle.

Damage to the abducens nerve often arises from stretching, if intracranial pressure rises in the compartments above the tentorium cerebelli. The patient then presents with a medial deviation of the affected eye and an inability to direct it laterally.

Cranial nerve VII – the facial nerve

(Fig. 3.51)

This complex cranial nerve has a number of functions:

1. it supplies the muscles of facial expression derived from the embryological second branchial arch (special visceral efferents)

2. it carries the parasympathetic secretomotor innervation to the submandibular and sublingual salivary glands and the palatine and lacrimal glands (general visceral efferents)
3. it carries taste sensation from the anterior two-thirds of the tongue (special visceral afferents)
4. it supplies the sensory innervation to much of the skin of the external auditory meatus, tympanic membrane and postauricular region (general somatic afferent).

The facial nerve appears at the lateral extensions of the pontomedullary junction as 2 roots: a larger medial root carrying the special visceral efferent fibers and a smaller, more laterally located nervus intermedius which carries all the other fibers (Fig. 3.42). Both roots pass laterally, in company with the vestibulocochlear nerve, to enter the internal auditory meatus on the posterior surface of the petrous temporal bone in the posterior cranial fossa. The nerve then traverses the canal for the facial nerve, which is directed laterally at first, and then passes forwards and superior to the vestibule of the inner ear. On reaching the wall which separates the middle from the inner ear, the canal turns abruptly backwards, forming the geniculum of the nerve. This is the location of the sensory geniculate

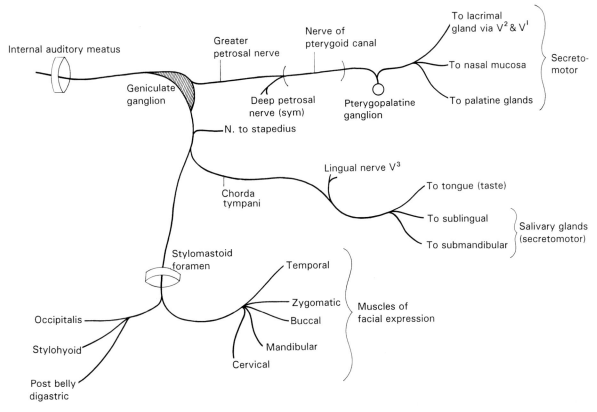

Fig. 3.51
Peripheral distribution of the facial nerve.

ganglion. On reaching the posterior wall of the tympanic cavity the canal turns inferiorly, running down to terminate at the stylomastoid foramen.

The special visceral efferent fibers arise from the motor nucleus of the facial nerve, which is situated in the caudal pontine tegmentum (Fig. 3.7). The fibers loop over the nucleus of the abducens nerve forming the facial colliculus in the floor of the fourth ventricle. These fibers follow the medial root described above and exit at the stylomastoid foramen to supply the muscles of the face, scalp and auricle as well as the buccinator, platysma, stylohyoid, posterior belly of digastric and stapedius muscles. The nerve to the stapedius muscle arises in the facial canal, distal to the geniculate ganglion. The posterior auricular nerve arises close to the exit of the facial nerve from the stylomastoid foramen, and passes upwards in front of the mastoid process and terminates in auricular and occipital branches. The former supplies the muscles of the auricle whilst the latter supplies the occipital region of the occipitofrontalis muscle. A digastric branch and a stylohyoid branch arise close to the stylomastoid foramen and supply the posterior belly of digastric and the stylohyoid muscles respectively. The facial nerve then winds lateral to the styloid process, the external carotid artery and the retromandibular vein in the cleft between the mastoid process and the external auditory meatus, before terminating in 5 branches. These terminal branches (temporal, zygomatic, buccal, mandibular and cervical) arise in the parotid salivary gland to supply the muscles of facial expression, buccinator and platysma. The cortical control of lower facial muscles is strictly contralateral but the muscles of the upper face have a bilateral cortical innervation. This is a useful fact for distinguishing between upper and lower motor neuron lesions.

The general visceral efferent fibers (parasympathetic secretomotor) arise from the superior salivatory nucleus and leave in the so-called nervus intermedius. Fibers reach the pterygopalatine ganglion via the greater petrosal nerve (which arises at the genu of the facial nerve) and the postganglionic fibers supply the lacrimal and palatine glands. Preganglionic fibers reach the submandibular ganglion via the chorda tympani nerve before synapsing and supplying the submandibular and sublingual salivary glands. The autonomic innervation to the head and neck will be considered in greater detail later (p. 146).

The special visceral afferent fibers arise from the taste buds on the anterior surface of the tongue. The fibers travel with the chorda tympani nerve and join with the facial nerve in the facial canal. The cell bodies of the primary sensory neurons are located in the geniculate ganglion, and the fibers enter the rostral part of the nucleus solitarius via the nervus intermedius.

The general somatic afferent fibers join the facial nerve via the vagal auricular branch and the cell bodies of these neurons are to be found in the geniculate ganglion. The fibers pass in the nervus intermedius to terminate in the spinal nucleus of the trigeminal nerve.

The long course of the facial nerve through a rigid bony canal makes it susceptible to compression should viral infection produce inflammation and swelling. Bell's palsy presents as a paralysis of the muscles of facial expression on the affected side, with asymmetry of the face, an inability to close the eye, and dribbling at the corner of the mouth with food collecting between the gums and cheek. Depending upon the location of the inflammation, there may also be a loss of taste in the anterior two-thirds of the tongue, dryness of the eye due to a reduction in tear production and a dry mouth due to a reduction in saliva. In addition, the patient may experience hyperacusis (increased sound perception) following paralysis of the stapedius muscle. Fractures of the base of the skull and pituitary tumors are also potential sources of damage to the facial nerve. In the newborn, the mastoid process is not formed and the stylomastoid foramen is vulnerable to damage from the vigorous application of forceps during delivery which will lead to facial paralysis on the damaged side only.

Supranuclear lesions, perhaps due to a cerebrovascular accident, will result in complete paralysis only of the facial muscles below the palpebral fissure. The patient will still be able to close the eyelids and wrinkle the forehead due to the bilateral innervation of the upper facial musculature.

Cranial nerve VIII – the vestibulocochlear nerve (Fig. 3.52)

This cranial nerve consists of 2 quite distinct parts: the vestibular nerve, which is concerned with balance, and the cochlear (auditory) nerve which is the nerve of hearing. Both are sensory nerves transmitting impulses from the internal ear.

The semicircular canals, utricle and saccule, are connected to the vestibular ganglia by short peripheral fibers. The vestibular nerve arises from the vestibular ganglia and passes medially within the petrous temporal bone to enter the skull at the internal auditory meatus. The nerve enters the medulla oblongata of the brainstem ventral to the inferior cerebellar peduncle. The central fibers then pass to the vestibular nuclei in the floor of the fourth ventricle although some fibers may bypass the nuclei to enter the cerebellum directly, via the inferior cerebellar peduncle. From the cerebellum, fibers pass to the spinal level via the vestibulospinal and reticulospinal pathways.

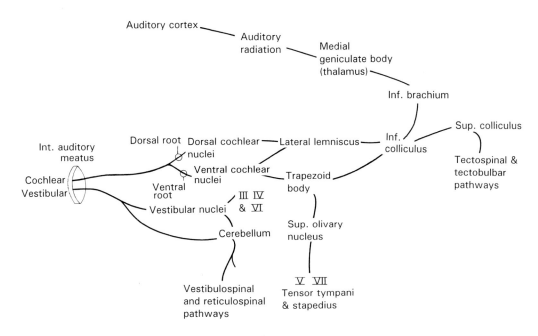

Fig. 3.52
Central connections of the vestibulocochlear nerve.

The cochlear nerve consists of central processes of bipolar cells in the spiral ganglion associated with the spiral organ of Corti. The cochlear nerve passes with the vestibular nerve to enter the intracranial region at the internal auditory meatus. The nerve passes medially and enters the medulla oblongata before dividing into a dorsal and a ventral root. The dorsal root passes to the dorsal cochlear nucleus in the lateral recess of the fourth ventricle, whilst the ventral root ends in the ventral cochlear nucleus on the inferior aspect of the inferior cerebellar peduncle. From the ventral nucleus, fibers decussate in the trapezoid body to reach the contralateral superior olivary nucleus. Fibers from the dorsal nucleus decussate and join efferents from the ventral nucleus to ascend in the lateral lemniscus. Fibers then relay in the inferior colliculus of the midbrain, traverse the inferior brachium and terminate in the medial geniculate body of the thalamus. Through the auditory radiation, the pathway reaches the auditory cortex of the temporal lobe. A reflex pathway involves fibers in the tectospinal and tectobulbar pathways through fibers that connect between the inferior and superior colliculi.

Disruption of auditory stimulation can occur anywhere along the pathway between the external auditory meatus and the auditory cortex. Damage to the vestibulocochlear nerve will result in a variety of symptoms, including varying degrees of hearing loss, tinnitus, nystagmus and vertigo.

Cranial nerve IX – the glossopharyngeal nerve (Fig. 3.53)

The glossopharyngeal nerve is a mixed nerve supplying the structures of the embryological third branchial arch. It carries branchiomotor (special visceral efferents) fibers which arise from the nucleus ambiguus and supply the stylopharyngeus muscle. Parasympathetic fibers (general visceral efferents) arise in the inferior salivatory nucleus and relay via the otic ganglion to supply both secretomotor and vasomotor fibers to the parotid salivary gland. Special visceral afferent (taste) fibers arise from the posterior one-third of the tongue and pass to the nucleus of the tractus solitarius. General visceral afferent fibers pass in the carotid branch of the glossopharyngeal nerve from the baroreceptors in the carotid sinus and chemoreceptors in the carotid body to the caudal region of the tractus solitarius. Pharyngeal nerves take part in the pharyngeal plexus with the vagus and cranial part of the accessory nerve to supply the mucosa of the middle ear, pharynx, soft palate, tonsil and posterior one-third of the tongue as well as the muscles of the soft palate (except the tensor veli palatini) and pharynx.

The glossopharyngeal nerve is located on the upper part of the medulla oblongata in the groove between the olive medially and the inferior cerebellar peduncle laterally (Fig. 3.42). It exits via a series of rootlets which are continuous below with the rootlets of the vagus and

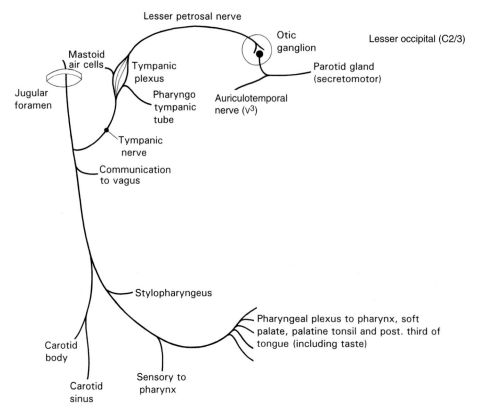

Fig. 3.53
Peripheral distribution of the glossopharyngeal nerve.

cranial accessory nerves. From here the nerve passes anteriorly and inferiorly, bending downwards at the petrous temporal bone before exiting from the skull via the jugular foramen. Below the skull, it passes anteriorly and inferiorly between the internal jugular vein and the internal carotid artery. Here it lies medial to the styloid process and the stylopharyngeus muscle. It then passes forwards between the superior and middle constrictor muscles of the pharynx ending in the branches which contribute to the pharyngeal plexus.

The glossopharyngeal nerve is deeply located and so is rarely damaged, although injury may lead to loss of the gag reflex, dysphagia, loss of taste in the posterior third of the tongue, decreased salivation and a loss of sensation on the affected side of the soft palate and pharynx.

Cranial nerve X – the vagus nerve
(Fig. 3.54)

This is one of the largest of the cranial nerves and has the widest distribution. It is the nerve supply to the fourth and sixth embryological branchial arches and as

such, carries branchiomotor fibers (special visceral efferents) which arise in the nucleus ambiguus to supply the muscles of the soft palate (except the tensor veli palatini), pharynx (except the stylopharyngeus), larynx and upper esophagus. Its parasympathetic component (general visceral efferents) arises from the dorsal vagal motor nucleus in the floor of the fourth ventricle and is visceromotor to the smooth muscle of the bronchi, esophagus, stomach, small intestine and the proximal two-thirds of the colon as well as the cardiac muscle. The vagal parasympathetic fibers are also secretomotor to the gastrointestinal glands and pancreas. Special visceral afferent fibers (taste) are limited to the small area around the epiglottis. It also carries a small number of general somatic afferent fibers which supply general sensation to the external auditory meatus and the dura mater of the posterior cranial fossa as well as the mucosa of the pharynx and larynx.

The vagus emerges from the lateral surface of the medulla oblongata by a series of rootlets that are continuous with those of the glossopharyngeal above and the cranial accessory below. The nerve passes out through the jugular foramen in a common dural sheath with the accessory nerve. The vagus has 2 ganglia

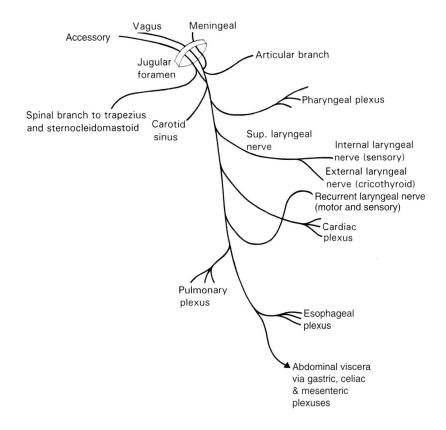

Fig. 3.54
Peripheral distribution of the vagus and accessory nerves.

within the jugular foramen – a small ganglion that houses the cell bodies of sensory fibers from the dura and external ear, and a much larger, more inferior, ganglion which is also sensory and contains the cell bodies of all the other afferent fibers.

The vagus emerges from the jugular foramen and lies within the carotid sheath between the internal jugular vein and the internal carotid artery. The cranial part of the accessory nerve fuses with the vagus in the region of the ganglia. The vagus continues inferiorly in the carotid sheath to the root of the neck. At the base of the skull the vagus gives off a meningeal branch which re-enters the skull to supply the dura mater of the posterior cranial fossa. The auricular branch also leaves the vagus close to its exit from the skull. It enters the mastoid canaliculus on the lateral wall of the jugular fossa, crosses the facial canal and then traverses the tympanomastoid fissure to supply some of the skin of the auricle, the posterior wall and floor of the external acoustic meatus, and the adjoining part of the outer surface of the tympanic membrane.

Within the neck, the vagus gives off the following branches:

1. **pharyngeal**, which enters the pharynx between the superior and middle constrictors to contribute to the pharyngeal plexus and thus supply the majority of the muscles of the soft palate, the superior and middle constrictors and the mucosa in the region of the palate.

2. The **superior laryngeal nerve**, which divides into 2 branches at the thyrohyoid membrane:
   — the **internal laryngeal nerve** pierces the membrane to supply sensation to the mucosa of the larynx down to the level of the vocal folds and it also carries the taste fibers from the epiglottis. The nerve passes close to the submucosal surface and so is easily blocked.
   — the **external laryngeal nerve** descends on the inferior constrictor, pierces and supplies it before terminating to supply the cricothyroid muscle.

3. Several **cardiac branches** arise in the neck and pass inferiorly to become incorporated into the cardiac plexus.

4. The **right recurrent laryngeal nerve** branches from the vagus as it passes anterior to the right subclavian artery. The right recurrent laryngeal nerve curves around the artery and ascends to lie lateral to the interval between the trachea anteriorly and the esophagus posteriorly. It then passes deep to the inferior constrictor to enter the larynx and supply all the muscles of the larynx except the cricothyroid

and is sensory to the mucosa below the level of the vocal folds.

The right and left nerves have a different course through the thorax. The **right vagus** passes anterior to the right subclavian artery and lies beneath the mediastinal pleura to the right of the trachea and posteromedial to the superior vena cava. The arch of the azygos vein comes between the nerve and the mediastinal pleura. Posterior to the root of the lung, the right vagus breaks up into several branches.

The **left vagus** enters the thorax between the left common carotid and left subclavian arteries, lying posterior to the left brachiocephalic vein. It descends deep to the mediastinal pleura and crosses the left side of the aortic arch before breaking up into several branches behind the root of the lung. The terminal branches of the vagus reunite to form the anterior and posterior vagal trunks, which pass into the abdomen through the esophageal opening. On reaching the anterior and posterior surfaces of the stomach, the anterior and posterior vagal trunks break up to form plexuses around the celiac and superior mesenteric arteries.

A number of branches pass from the vagus within the thorax. These are:

1. The **left recurrent laryngeal nerve**, which leaves the vagus on the lateral surface of the aortic arch and winds around the arch to lie posterior to the ligamentum arteriosum. It then ascends in the interval between the trachea anteriorly and the esophagus posteriorly and has the same distribution as the right recurrent laryngeal nerve.
2. Further **cardiac branches** arise in the thoracic region and become incorporated into the cardiac plexus.
3. **Pulmonary branches** become incorporated into the pulmonary plexus.
4. **Esophageal branches** supply the muscular coat and mucosa of the esophagus.

Damage to the vagus nerve is rare but a unilateral lesion of the nerve will produce sagging of the soft palate, hoarseness due to paralysis of the vocal cords and dysphagia. Complex reflexes associated with the vagus are difficult to explain fully but, for example, a plug of wax or a foreign object which becomes lodged in the external auditory canal can provoke a persistent cough. Syringing the meatus may cause vomiting or coughing and, in very rare cases, vagal inhibition of the heart and sudden death.

Cranial nerve XI – the accessory nerve (Fig. 3.54)

The accessory nerve originates from both a smaller cranial and a larger spinal root. The cranial root arises from the lateral surface of the medulla oblongata in line with the vagus nerve and is branchiomotor in origin (Fig. 3.42). The spinal root arises from the first 5 cervical segments of the spinal cord, where the nerve roots emerge between the ventral and dorsal spinal nerve roots, and ascends posterior to the ligamentum denticulum. The spinal root enters the posterior cranial fossa via the foramen magnum behind the vertebral artery where it joins with the cranial root. The united accessory nerve passes out though the jugular foramen before splitting again into cranial and spinal components. The fibers of **cranial** origin are distributed with the pharyngeal and laryngeal branches of the vagus nerve to supply muscles of the soft palate, pharynx and larynx as described above. The fibers of **spinal** origin descend into the neck and cross the transverse process of the atlas before being crossed by the occipital artery. The nerve then descends obliquely, medial to the styloid process and deep to the sternocleidomastoid muscle, which it supplies. In the posterior triangle of the neck it lies on the levator scapulae muscle, being closely related to the superficial cervical lymph nodes, and then passes into the trapezius muscle, which it supplies. It is said that the innervation to the sternocleidomastoid is ipsilateral, whilst that to the trapezius is contralateral.

Damage to the accessory nerve usually occurs either at the point of exit from the jugular foramen as a result of a cranial base fracture or in the posterior triangle. The most obvious result of a lower lesion is a torticollis with paralysis and atrophy of the affected muscles.

Cranial nerve XII – the hypoglossal nerve (Fig. 3.55)

The twelfth cranial nerve is a somatic efferent nerve that supplies all the intrinsic muscles of the tongue as well as the extrinsic styloglossus, hyoglossus and genioglossus. The hypoglossal nerve exits from the medulla oblongata as a series of rootlets in the groove posterior to the pyramid and anterior to the olive (Fig. 3.42). The nerve exits from the skull via the hypoglossal canal, which can be bifid due to the presence of a

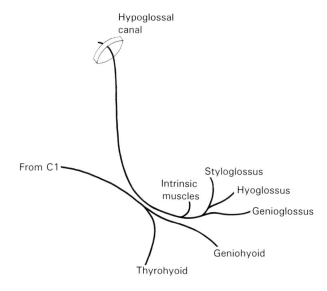

Fig. 3.55
Peripheral distribution of the hypoglossal nerve.

hypoglossal ponticle. The nerve then descends almost vertically behind the glossopharyngeal and vagus nerves to occupy a position between the internal jugular vein and the internal carotid artery. It then descends to the level of the angle of the mandible, loops around the sternocleidomastoid branch of the occipital artery and crosses the loop of the lingual artery above the tip of the greater horn of the hyoid bone before running forwards on the hyoglossus muscle.

A supranuclear lesion results in a contralateral weakness with limited evidence of muscle atrophy. As the supply to genioglossus is wholly contralateral, when the tongue is protruded it deviates to the opposite side from which the lesion has occurred. However, in infranuclear lesions there is obvious atrophy of half of the tongue and, when protruded, it deviates to the side of the lesion.

THE CRANIAL NERVES

I	**Olfactory**	
	Special somatic afferent	Smell
II	**Optic**	
	Special somatic afferent	Vision
III	**Oculomotor**	
	General somatic efferent	Extra-ocular muscles except superior oblique and lateral rectus
	General visceral efferent	Sphincter pupillae and ciliary muscle
IV	**Trochlear**	
	General somatic efferent	Superior oblique muscle
V	**Trigeminal**	
	General somatic afferent	Face, scalp, mouth, teeth, nasal cavity and air sinuses
	Special visceral efferent	Muscles of mastication, tensor tympani and tensor veli palatini
VI	**Abducens**	
	General somatic efferent	Lateral rectus
VII	**Facial**	
	General somatic afferent	External auditory meatus, tympanic membrane and postauricular skin
	Special visceral afferent	Taste from anterior 2/3 tongue, soft palate and palatal arches
	General visceral efferent	Secretomotor to submandibular and sublingual salivary glands, palatine and lacrimal glands
	Special visceral efferent	Muscles of facial expression, platysma, stylohyoid, posterior belly of digastric and stapedius
VIII	**Vestibulocochlear**	
	Special somatic afferent	Equilibration and hearing
IX	**Glossopharyngeal**	
	General somatic afferent	Middle ear, mastoid air cells, pharyngotympanic tube and posterior 1/3 tongue
	General visceral afferent	Carotid sinus and carotid body
	Special visceral afferent	Taste from posterior 1/3 tongue
	General visceral efferent	Parotid salivary gland
	Special visceral efferent	Via plexus, to muscles of pharynx, soft palate, tonsil, posterior 1/3 of the tongue and stylopharyngeus

THE CRANIAL NERVES (Contd.)

X	**Vagus**	
	General somatic afferent	External auditory meatus, tympanic membrane, auricle, pharynx and dura mater
	General visceral afferent	Aortic arch
	Special visceral afferent	Region of epiglottis
	General visceral efferent	Smooth muscle of bronchi, esophagus, stomach, small intestine, proximal 2/3 colon, cardiac muscle, gastro-intestinal glands and pancreas
	Special visceral efferent	Muscles of soft palate, pharynx, larynx and upper esophagus
XI	**Accessory**	
	Special visceral efferent	Soft palate, pharynx, larynx (sternocleidomastoid and trapezius)
XII	**Hypoglossal**	
	General somatic efferent	All intrinsic lingual muscles, styloglossus, hyoglossus and genioglossus

SPINAL CORD

The spinal cord lies within the vertebral canal and extends from the medulla oblongata above to the conus medullaris below (Fig. 3.56). At 12 fetal weeks the vertebral column and spinal cord are of a similar length, but due to the rapid growth of the bony column, the spinal cord only extends as far as L3 at birth and in the adult to around the lower border of the first lumbar vertebra. Therefore, in the adult, the spinal

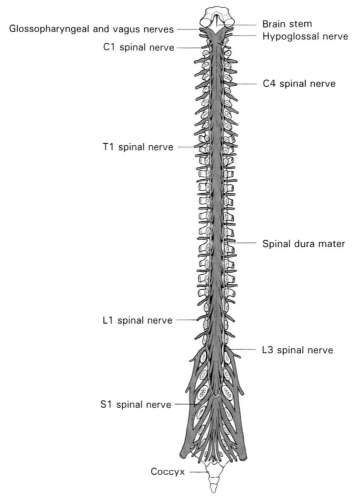

Glossopharyngeal and vagus nerves

Brain stem

Hypoglossal nerve

C1 spinal nerve

C4 spinal nerve

T1 spinal nerve

Spinal dura mater

L1 spinal nerve

L3 spinal nerve

S1 spinal nerve

Coccyx

Fig. 3.56
The spinal cord within the vertebral canal.

segments tend to be located somewhat cranial to the vertebrae of the corresponding number so that, for example, the spinal segment of T1 lies opposite the C7 vertebra, the L1 segment opposite the T11 vertebra and the S5 segment opposite the L1 vertebra. This cranial displacement of the spinal cord segments results in a lengthening of the lower spinal nerves to enable them to reach their appropriate exit point from the vertebral column. This is the cauda equina which extends from the mid-lumbar region of the vertebral column to the termination of the spinal meninges at the S2 level (Fig. 3.57). The spinal cord tapers into a slender filament called the filum terminale, which lies in the midst of the cauda equina and terminates in the dorsal region of the coccyx.

Each spinal segment gives rise to 1 pair of spinal nerves, so that there are normally 31 pairs (8 cervical, 12 thoracic, 5 lumbar, 5 sacral and 1 coccygeal). However, due to the resegmentation process of the

sclerotome during embryological development of the vertebral column, only 7 cervical vertebrae survive. Therefore the first 7 spinal nerves exit from the cord cranial to the vertebra of the corresponding number but the remainder exit caudad to the vertebra of the corresponding number with the C8 exiting between the C7 and the T1 vertebrae.

The spinal cord is neither uniform in shape nor size throughout its length and presents 2 enlargements in the cervical (C4–T1) and lumbar (L1–S3) regions for the innervation of the upper and lower limbs respectively. The diameter of the spinal cord is greatest in the cervical region, as the amount of white matter decreases in a caudal direction. This explains the relatively large dimensions of the vertebral canal in the cervical compared with the lumbar vertebrae.

A ventral median fissure extends throughout the length of the ventral aspect of the cord. It is filled by the linea splendens of the pia mater and is the location

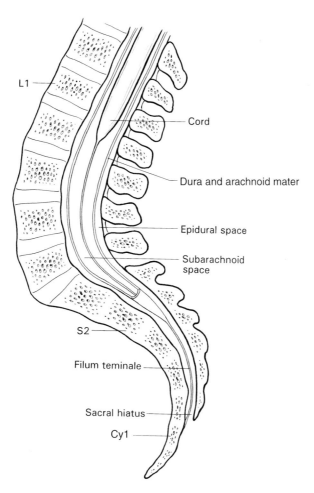

L1

Cord

Dura and arachnoid mater

Epidural space

Subarachnoid space

S2

Filum teminale

Sacral hiatus

Cy1

Fig. 3.57
Sagittal section to show the lower limits of the spinal cord and meninges

of the anterior spinal artery (Fig. 3.58). The corresponding dorsal median fissure is very shallow, as is the ventrolateral sulcus, which is the position of the attachment of the ventral roots of the spinal nerves. The dorsolateral sulcus marks the site of attachment of the dorsal spinal nerve roots.

Gray matter

On transverse section, the gray matter of the cord is located medially and is roughly 'H'-shaped being surrounded by 3 columns or funiculi of white matter (Fig. 3.58). The gray matter encloses the small spinal canal, which is the remnant of the central canal of the neural tube and is located in the region of the gray commissure which connects the right and left sides of the cord. On each side, the gray matter is elongated into dorsal and ventral horns and an intermediate lateral horn is found in cord segments T1–L2. The gray matter is an accumulation of neuronal cell bodies

a. the dorsal horn – predominantly sensory in function and arranged into 4 discrete columns (substantia gelatinosa, nucleus proprius, thoracic nucleus and visceral afferent nucleus)
b. the lateral horn – visceral efferent in function, and
c. the ventral horn – predominantly somatomotor in function (Fig. 3.59).

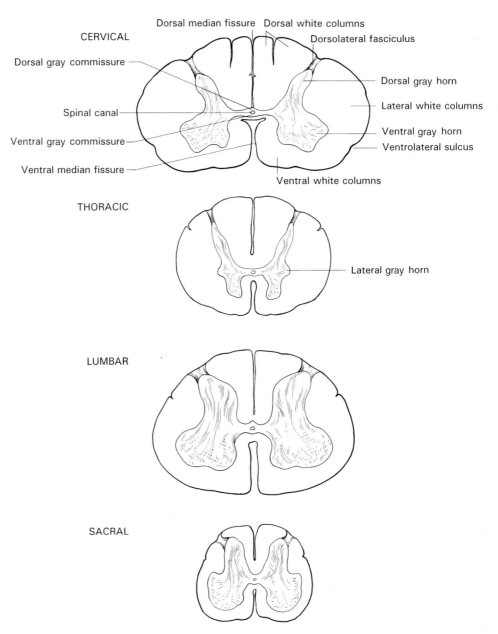

Fig. 3.58
Variation in shape of the spinal cord at different vertebral levels.

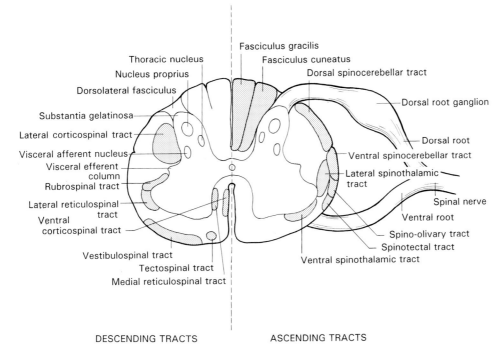

DESCRIPTIVE TRACTS   ASCENDING TRACTS

Fig. 3.59
Some of the major tracts and nuclei in the spinal cord.

The spinal cord segments are not consistent in length, with the lumbar and sacral segments being considerably shorter, so that the amount of gray matter appears greater in this region. The amount of gray matter increases considerably in the region of the cervical and lumbar enlargements.

White matter

The white matter of the cord represents the axons or tracts of the neurons whose cell bodies can be found in gray matter. There are 3 funiculi or columns (Fig. 3.59):

  a. the ventral funiculus between the ventral median fissure and the ventral roots of the spinal nerves
  b. the lateral funiculus between the dorsal and ventral spinal roots
  c. the dorsal funiculus between the dorsal roots of the spinal nerves and the dorsal median septum.

The white matter consists of tracts that both ascend from lower to higher centers and descend from higher to lower centers. Figure 3.59 shows the location of some of the more important tracts with the ascending tracts on the right of the diagram and the descending tracts on the left. The ascending tracts that carry pain and temperature (lateral spinothalamic tract), light touch and pressure (ventral spinothalamic tract) and conscious proprioception, vibration and discriminative touch (dorsal columns) from the body wall and limbs are a 3-neuron contralateral pathway where the fibers will relay in the thalamus before passing to the appropriate region of the cerebral cortex. Ascending

tracts that pass to the cerebellum (dorsal and ventral spinocerebellar and cuneocerebellar) are a 2-neuron ipsilateral pathway. Other more minor ascending tracts are the spino-olivary, spinoreticular, spinotectal and propriospinal pathways.

The descending tracts are grouped into 2 systems:

1. The **pyramidal system** comprises those motor fibers that synapse either in the motor nuclei of cranial nerves (corticonuclear/bulbar pathway) or on ventral horn cells of the spinal cord (ventral and lateral corticospinal pathways). In this way, the motor innervation to striated muscle is achieved through lower motor neurons in both the cranial and spinal nerves.
2. The **extrapyramidal system** comprises all other descending tracts (e.g. vestibulospinal, reticulospinal, rubrospinal and tectospinal).

The extrapyramidal pathways are phylogenetically older and represent a more diverse and complex motor system, being concerned predominantly with locomotion, posture and gross movements of the trunk and head. Conversely, the pyramidal system is phylogenetically more recent and controls fine, skilled, motor-related activities.

Arterial supply and venous drainage of the spinal cord

The arterial supply to the spinal cord is derived from the anterior and posterior spinal arteries with segmental back-up from spinal branches of the vertebral, deep cervical, intercostal and lumbar arteries (Fig. 3.60).

As each **vertebral artery** nears its termination, it gives off a small branch which passes down the ventral surface of the medulla oblongata and eventually fuses with its partner from the opposite side to form the **anterior spinal artery**. This descends through the foramen magnum and runs the full length of the spinal cord, occupying the ventral median fissure. Central branches pass from the anterior spinal artery into the cord and supply the anterior gray column, the base of the dorsal gray column and adjacent white matter. The blood supply to the spinal cord is readily compromised due to the absence of a collateral circulation.

The **posterior spinal arteries** can also branch from the vertebral arteries but they more commonly arise from the inferior cerebellar arteries. They descend through the foramen magnum as 2 branches which

pass one in front of, and one behind, the dorsal roots of the spinal nerves.

At regular intervals these arteries are supported by a series of paired **radicular arteries** which are derived from various spinal branches of segmental arteries. The radicular arteries pass along the ventral and dorsal roots of the spinal nerves (Fig. 3.61). The ventral radiculars are small and often terminate along the ventral root or in the arterial plexus of the pia mater. The dorsal radiculars are larger and supply the region of the dorsal root ganglion and the remainder of the dorsal gray matter before synapsing with branches of the anterior spinal artery. One large ventral radicular artery (arteria radicularis magna) generally arises in the lower thoracic and lumbar region and usually on the left-hand side. Upon reaching the spinal cord it bifurcates into 2 branches: one that anastomoses with the anterior spinal artery and one that anastomoses

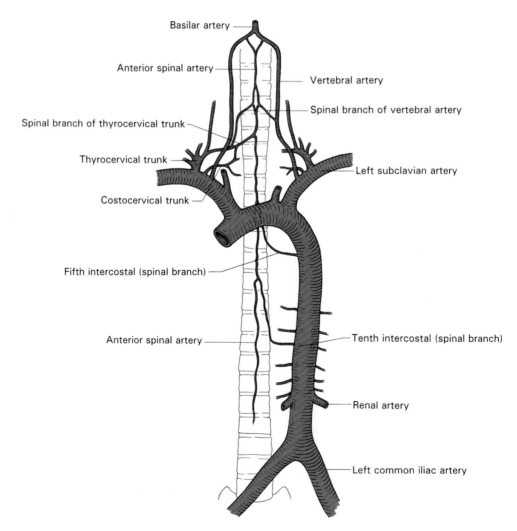

Fig. 3.60
The anterior spinal artery (with the aorta displaced laterally to show appropriate branches).

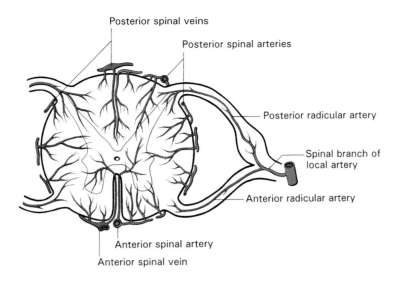

Fig. 3.61
The blood supply of the spinal cord.

with the posterior spinal artery. It is often large enough to supply almost two-thirds of the lower region of the spinal cord.

The anastomoses between the anterior and posterior spinal arteries, the radicular arteries and the arteria radicularis magna are complex and form longitudinal arterial channels that run the length of the spinal column. These channels are not always continuous and show considerable individual variation.

Venous drainage of the spinal cord is via 6 tortuous channels. Singular **anterior** and **posterior median longitudinal veins** run in their appropriate fissures whilst paired **anterolateral** and **posterolateral veins** run anterior and posterior to both the ventral and

dorsal spinal nerve roots. Ultimate drainage is either superiorly into the inferior cerebellar veins and inferior petrosal sinus or via intervertebral veins into the posterior intercostal, vertebral, lumbar and lateral sacral veins.

SPINAL NERVES

Each spinal nerve is formed from the fusion of ventral and dorsal roots and so is generally referred to as a mixed nerve as it carries both sensory and motor information (Fig. 3.62). These nerves are specific to segmental dermatomes and myotomes and a single

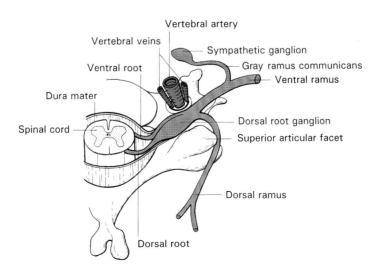

Fig. 3.62
The course of a typical cervical nerve in relation to its vertebra.

pair arises from each segment of the spinal cord. Therefore there are 8 cervical, 12 thoracic, 5 lumbar, 5 sacral and 1 coccygeal, forming a total of 31 pairs of spinal nerves. These exit from the vertebral canal via an intervertebral foramen which is formed from the upper and lower boundaries of the pedicles of adjacent vertebrae.

The **dorsal root** of a spinal nerve comprises the central processes of primary afferent neurons that pass from a sensory receptor towards the dorsal gray matter of the spinal cord. The cell bodies of these neurons are located in the paravertebral dorsal root ganglia (Fig. 3.62) and their axons pass medially to eventually synapse with a secondary neuron in the gray matter of the central nervous system. The **ventral root** of a spinal nerve comprises the efferent axons of lower motor neurons whose cell bodies are located in the ventral gray matter of the spinal cord. The ventral and dorsal roots fuse, and then shortly after they emerge from the intervertebral foramina divide into 4 branches – meningeal recurrent, rami communicantes, dorsal and ventral rami.

The **meningeal recurrent branch** is small and supplies the vertebrae, spinal meninges and the associated blood vessels. The **rami communicantes** are the general visceral efferent and afferent pathways

which will be considered with the autonomic nervous system (page 146).

Dorsal rami

The dorsal rami of the spinal nerves are usually smaller than their ventral counterparts. As a general rule, all dorsal rami separate into medial and lateral branches (with the exception of C1, S4–Cy1) with all branches supplying deep posterior muscles of the neck and back and only either the medial or the lateral branch reaching the skin to supply sensory innervation (Figs 3.63 and 3.64).

The dorsal ramus of **C1** is considerably larger than the ventral ramus and is generally known as the **suboccipital nerve**, as it passes through the suboccipital triangle to supply the muscles of this region (rectus capitis posterior major and minor, semispinalis capitis and the superior and inferior obliques). The dorsal ramus of C1 does not generally reach as far as the skin. A small filament passes from the branch to the inferior oblique muscle to join the C2 dorsal ramus.

The dorsal ramus of the **C2** spinal nerve is slightly larger than its corresponding ventral ramus and exits

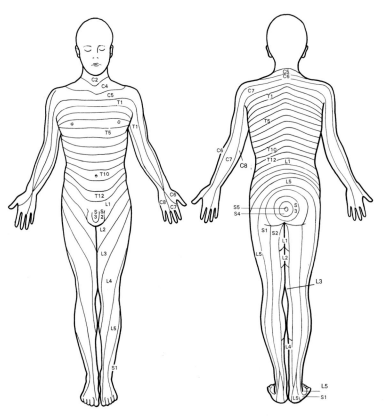

Fig. 3.63
The dermatomes.

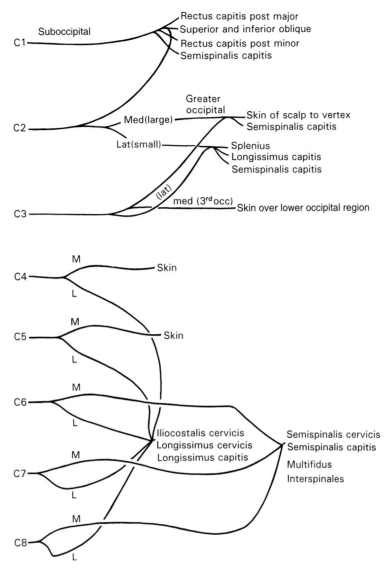

Fig. 3.64
The dorsal rami of the cervical nerves.

from the vertebral canal inferior to the posterior arch of the atlas but superior to the lamina of the axis. It passes a connecting filament to the C1 dorsal ramus before bifurcating into a larger medial branch and a much smaller lateral branch. The medial branch, which is also known as the **greater occipital nerve**, receives a small communicating filament from the medial branch of the C3 dorsal root. The greater occipital nerve is cutaneous to the scalp up to the vertex; it also supplies the semispinalis capitis muscle (Fig. 3.65). The smaller lateral branch is joined by the lateral branch of the C3 dorsal ramus and supplies the deep muscles of the neck including the splenius capitis, longissimus capitis and semispinalis capitis muscles.

The dorsal ramus of the **C3** spinal nerve also divides into medial and lateral branches, with the latter joining the lateral branch of the C2 dorsal ramus. The medial branch sends a small filament which connects with the medial branch of the C2 nerve but the larger proportion of this branch continues as the **third cervical nerve** to supply the skin of the lower occipital region.

The dorsal rami of the remainder of the cervical nerves (C4–C8) all bifurcate into medial and lateral branches. Generally only the medial branches of C4 and C5 reach the skin over the lower aspect of the neck, whereas all the other terminations innervate the deep muscles of the neck, including the iliocostalis cervicis, longissimus cervicis, longissimus capitis, semispinalis cervicis, multifidus, interspinales, etc.

All the dorsal rami of the **thoracic** spinal nerves bifurcate into medial and lateral branches. The medial

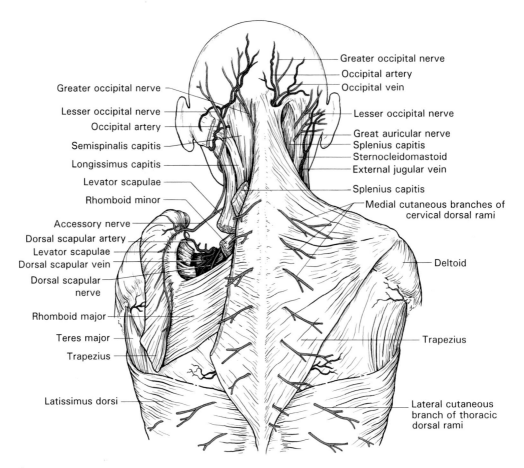

Fig. 3.65
The nerves and vessels of the upper back and posterior neck.

branches of nerves T1–T6 supply the skin and the semispinalis thoracis and multifidus muscles, whilst the medial branches of nerves T7–T12 only supply the overlying deep muscles and do not reach the skin. The lateral branches of T1–T6 supply the overlapping deep muscles of the back whilst it is the lateral branches of T7–T12 that pass to the skin. The dermatomes supplied by the dorsal rami of the thoracic nerves follow the obliquity of the ribs, so that the upper dermatomes are more horizontal whilst the lower dermatomes adopt a more oblique path (Fig. 3.66).

The dorsal rami of the **lumbar** nerves also all bifurcate into medial and lateral branches. All medial branches supply the multifidus muscle, whilst the lateral branches supply the sacrospinalis muscle, and only the terminal branches of L1–L3 reach the skin to supply the region over the superior posterolateral gluteal region.

Only the dorsal rami of S1–S3 bifurcate into medial and lateral branches and again the former supplies the multifidus muscle. The lateral branches form a loop on the dorsal aspect of the sacrum and join with L5 and S4 components to supply the remainder of the skin over the gluteal region.

The dorsal rami of the S4–S5 and Cy1 nerves do not divide but form a loop to supply the skin over the region of the coccyx.

Ventral rami

The ventral rami of the spinal nerves are usually larger than their corresponding dorsal rami and supply the limbs and anterolateral aspects of the trunk. It is only in the thoracic region that the ventral rami are independent of each other, due to the intervention of the ribs; in the cervical, lumbar and sacral regions adjacent ventral rami unite near their origins forming nerve plexuses – cervical, brachial and lumbosacral.

Cervical plexus

The ventral rami of C1–C4 form the **cervical plexus** and, in summary, are responsible for the innervation of the skin of the head, neck and upper chest and the innervation of the muscles of the neck and the diaphragm (Fig. 3.67). Each ramus, with the exception of C1, divides into ascending and descending parts which unite adjacent rami by communication loops. These divisions then separate into superficial and deep sets of nerves, with the former supplying the skin by ascending and descending branches and the latter supplying muscles through medial and lateral terminations. In addition, there are communications

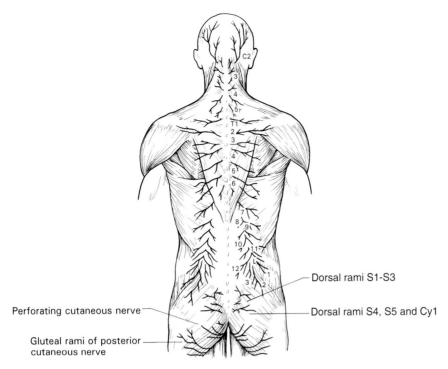

Fig. 3.66
Cutaneous distribution of the dorsal rami of the spinal nerves.

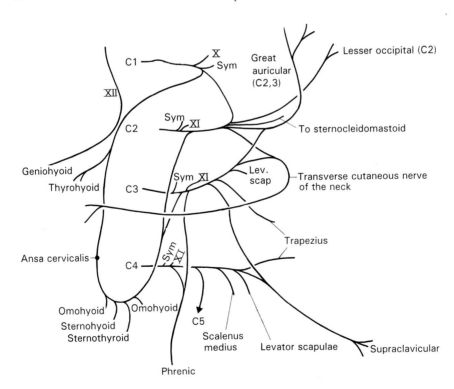

Fig. 3.67
The cervical plexus.

between C1–C4 and the vagus, accessory and hypoglossal nerves as well as gray rami communicantes from the superior sympathetic cervical ganglion. Although Figure 3.67 shows the cervical plexus, the pattern of distribution is better understood in functional rather than topographical terms.

BRANCHES OF THE CERVICAL PLEXUS

Superficial ascending (sensory)

Lesser occipital nerve (C2)
Greater auricular nerve (C2–C3)
Transverse cutaneous nerve of the neck (C2–C3)

Superficial descending (sensory)

Supraclavicular nerves (C3–C4)

Deep – medial branches (motor)

Communicating	Vagus(C1–C2)
	Hypoglossal (C1–C2)
	Sympathetic (C1–C4)
Muscular	Rectus capitis lateralis (C1)
	Rectus capitis anterior (C1–C2)
	Longus capitis (C1–C3)
	Longus colli (C2–C4)
	Phrenic nerve (C3–C5)

Deep – lateral branches (motor)

Communicating	Accessory (C2–C4)
Muscular	Sternocleidomastoid (C2–C3)
	Trapezius (C3–C4)
	Levator scapulae (C3–C4)
	Scalenus medius (C3–C4)

Ansa cervicalis

Geniohyoid and thyrohyoid (C1 through the hypoglossal nerve)
Omohyoid, sternohyoid and sternothyroid (C2–C3)

Superficial ascending branches
The **lesser occipital nerve** is predominantly formed from the C2 root, although some fibers can arise from C3 (Fig. 3.68). It passes around the accessory nerve and ascends along the posterior border of the sternocleidomastoid muscle. It then passes behind the auricle to supply the posterior part of the neck below the superior nuchal line. It communicates with the greater auricular nerve, the greater occipital nerve and the posterior auricular branch of the facial nerve. A small auricular branch may supply the upper third of the auricle, although this is usually derived from the greater occipital nerve.

The **greater auricular nerve** is the largest of the ascending branches and carries fibers from both the C2 and C3 spinal nerves. It encircles the posterior border of the sternocleidomastoid muscle, below the level of the lesser occipital nerve, and ascends on this muscle in company with the external jugular vein. In the region of the parotid gland it divides into anterior and posterior branches. The anterior branch supplies the skin of the face over the region of the parotid gland, whilst the posterior branch supplies the skin over the mastoid process and the posterior aspect of the auricle. It communicates with the lesser occipital nerve, the auricular branch of the vagus and the posterior auricular branch of the facial nerve.

The **transverse cutaneous nerve** of the neck arises from the C2 and C3 roots. It appears at the posterior border of the sternocleidomastoid muscle below the

level of the greater auricular nerve and runs forwards deep to the external jugular vein. It passes to the anterior border of the sternocleidomastoid muscle and divides into an ascending and a descending branch. The former passes to the submandibular region to supply the skin of the upper region of the front of the neck. The descending branch pierces platysma and supplies the skin of the side and front of the neck as far inferiorly as the sternum. This nerve is therefore responsible for the sensory innervation to the front of the neck from the chin to the sternum.

Superficial descending branches
The **supraclavicular nerves** arise as a common trunk from the C3 and C4 roots. They emerge, in common with the 3 preceding nerves, at the posterior border of the sternocleidomastoid muscle and divide into 3 groups of nerves:

1. Medial (suprasternal), which cross the external jugular vein to supply the midline skin as far inferiorly as the manubriosternal angle.
2. Intermediate (supraclavicular nerves proper), which cross the clavicle to supply the skin over the pectoralis major and deltoid muscles down to the level of the second rib.
3. Lateral (supra-acromial), which cross the trapezius muscle and acromion process of the scapula to supply the skin over the upper and posterior regions of the shoulder.

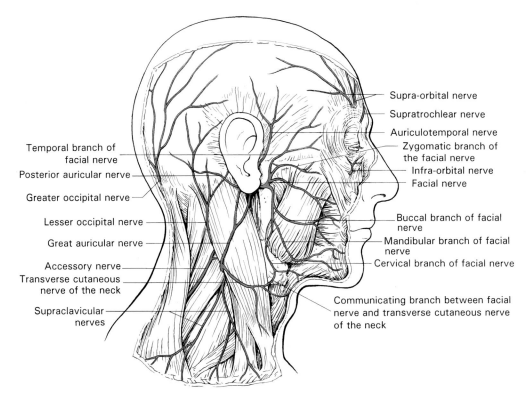

Fig. 3.68
The nerves of the scalp, face and neck.

Deep medial branches

The **communicating** branches are several small twigs that connect with the vagus nerve (C1–C2), the hypoglossal nerve (C1) and the superior cervical sympathetic ganglion (C1–C4). The branch from C1 travels with the hypoglossal nerve for a short distance before separating as the superior root of the ansa cervicalis and carrying the nerve supply to the thyrohyoid and geniohyoid muscles.

The **muscular** branches supply the rectus capitis lateralis, rectus capitis anterior, longus capitis and longus colli muscles.

The **phrenic** nerve is the sole motor supply to the thoracic diaphragm. It arises principally from the C4 root but also carries some fibers from the C3 and C5 nerves. It forms at the lateral border of the scalenus anterior muscle and runs vertically across the front of that muscle, passing deep to the sternocleidomastoid and inferior belly of the omohyoid muscle, internal jugular vein, transverse cutaneous and suprascapular arteries. It enters the thorax via the thoracic inlet in front of the internal thoracic artery between the subclavian artery and vein. An accessory phrenic nerve may arise from the C5 contribution, frequently from the branch to the subclavius muscle. It lies lateral to the main nerve and usually joins it around the level of the first rib, although it can remain separate as far inferiorly as the root of the lung.

Deep lateral branches

The **communicating** branches are associated with the accessory cranial nerve (C2–C4) and pass through the substance of the sternocleidomastoid muscle.

The **muscular** branches are distributed to the sternocleidomastoid, trapezius, levator scapulae and scalenus medius muscles with the fibers to the two former muscles being predominantly proprioceptive in nature.

Ansa cervicalis

This is almost an accessory cervical plexus supplying the infrahyoid strap muscles and the geniohyoid muscle (Fig. 3.67). The superior root of the ansa arises from the C1 root and runs for a short distance with the hypoglossal nerve before bifurcating into a branch which passes to the thyrohyoid and geniohyoid muscles and a descending branch which eventually joins up with the inferior root of the ansa. This inferior root (nervus descendens cervicalis) is formed from the C2 and C3 roots and passes lateral to the internal jugular vein before joining the superior root of the ansa in front of the common carotid artery. Branches arise from the loop of the ansa to supply the sternohyoid and sternothyroid muscles and both bellies of the omohyoid muscle.

128 | ## Brachial plexus

The brachial plexus is formed from the ventral rami of spinal nerves C5–T1 (Fig. 3.69). In what is termed a prefixed plexus there is also a large contribution from the C4 ramus whilst the T1 component is reduced. Conversely, in the more usual postfixed plexus the contribution from C4 is small, that from T1 is large and there is always a T2 contribution in the form of the intercostobrachial nerve. The brachial plexus is the basis of the musculocutaneous innervation of the upper limb. The **roots** of the plexus pass out through the appropriate intervertebral foramina and are situated predominantly in the posterior triangle of the neck (Fig. 3.70). The roots of the C5 and C6 ventral rami combine at the lateral border of the scalenus medius muscle to form the **upper trunk** of the brachial plexus. The roots of the C8 and T1 rami unite behind the scalenus anterior muscle to form the **lower trunk**, whilst the C7 root does not combine and continues as the **middle trunk** of the plexus. The trunks descend laterally and pass above and behind the clavicle where each splits into an anterior and a posterior division. Upon emerging from the lower border of the clavicle the anterior divisions of the upper and middle trunks have united to form the **lateral cord** of the brachial plexus whilst the anterior division of the lower trunk has become the **medial cord** of the brachial plexus. All 3 posterior divisions from each trunk unite to form the

posterior cord of the brachial plexus. Within the axilla, the three cords adopt their respective positions medial, lateral and posterior to the axillary artery.

The branches of the brachial plexus are either supra- or infraclavicular as there are no branches from the divisions of the plexus as it passes behind the clavicle.

Supraclavicular branches

The terminal branches that arise from the roots of the brachial plexus are as follows:

1. Branches to the scaleni and longus colli muscles which arise from the C5–C8 components close to the point of exit from the appropriate intervertebral foramen.
2. A branch from C5 that passes with the phrenic nerve (C3–C5).
3. The **dorsal scapular nerve** (C5), which runs with the deep branch of the dorsal scapular artery to supply the rhomboid minor and major muscles.
4. The **long thoracic nerve** (C5–C7), which descends dorsal to the brachial plexus to reach the serratus anterior muscle.

The terminal branches that arise from the upper trunk of the brachial plexus are as follows:

1. The **nerve to subclavius** (C5–C6), which supplies the muscle of the same name.
2. The **suprascapular nerve** (C5–C6), which is a large

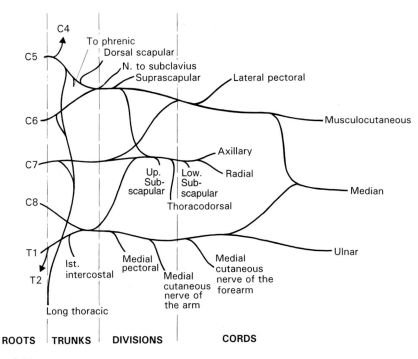

Fig. 3.69
The brachial plexus.

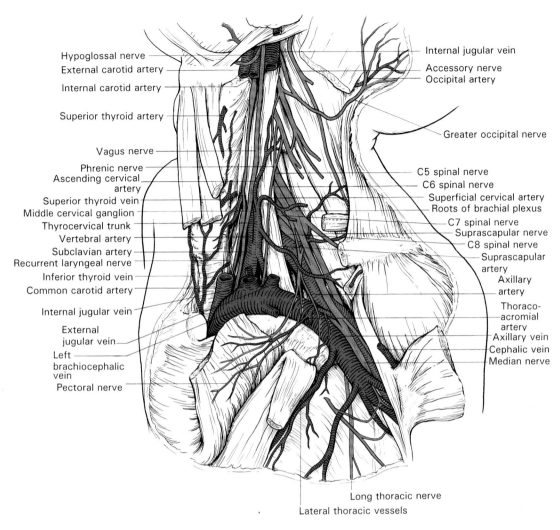

Hypoglossal nerve
External carotid artery
Internal carotid artery
Superior thyroid artery
Vagus nerve
Phrenic nerve
Ascending cervical artery
Superior thyroid vein
Middle cervical ganglion
Thyrocervical trunk
Vertebral artery
Subclavian artery
Recurrent laryngeal nerve
Inferior thyroid vein
Common carotid artery
Internal jugular vein
External jugular vein
Left brachiocephalic vein
Pectoral nerve

Internal jugular vein
Accessory nerve
Occipital artery
Greater occipital nerve
C5 spinal nerve
C6 spinal nerve
Superficial cervical artery
Roots of brachial plexus
C7 spinal nerve
Suprascapular nerve
C8 spinal nerve
Suprascapular artery
Axillary artery
Thoraco-acromial artery
Axillary vein
Cephalic vein
Median nerve

Long thoracic nerve
Lateral thoracic vessels

Fig. 3.70
The root of the neck.

branch that passes deep to the trapezius and omohyoid muscles to enter the supraspinous fossa under the transverse scapular ligament. It supplies the supraspinatus muscle and then enters the infraspinous fossa to supply the infraspinatus muscle by curving around the lateral border of the scapular spine with the suprascapular artery. It also sends articular twigs to both the shoulder and the acromioclavicular joints.

Infraclavicular branches

The terminal branches that arise from the infraclavicular portion of the brachial plexus all originate from the cords.

Lateral cord

There are 3 terminal branches from the lateral cord of the brachial plexus and the fibers originate from the anterior divisions of the C5–C7 roots:

1. The **lateral pectoral nerve** (C5–C7) crosses anterior to the axillary vessels and is distributed to the deep surface of the pectoralis major muscle. Some fibers are passed on to the medial pectoral nerve to supply the pectoralis minor muscle.
2. The **musculocutaneous nerve** (C5–C7) arises opposite the lower border of the pectoralis minor muscle (Fig. 3.71). It passes downwards and laterally between the biceps brachii and brachialis to reach the lateral side of the arm where it continues into the forearm as the **lateral cutaneous nerve of the forearm**. On its course through the arm it supplies the coracobrachialis, both heads of biceps brachii, most of the brachialis and some branches to the elbow joint. The surface markings of the nerve pass in a line drawn distally from the lateral side of the third part of the axillary artery and laterally across the elevations produced by the coracobrachialis and the biceps brachii to the lateral side of the insertion of the biceps tendon.

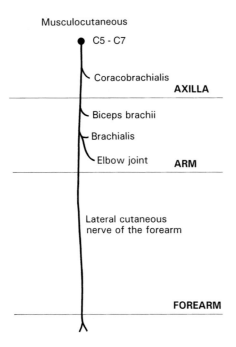

Fig. 3.71
The distribution of the musculocutaneous nerve.

3. The lateral root of the **median nerve** (C6–C7) joins with the medial root from the medial cord, anterior to the axillary artery (Figs 3.72 and 3.73).

Medial cord
There are 5 terminal branches from the medial cord of the brachial plexus and the fibers originate from the anterior divisions of the C8 and T1 roots:

1. The **medial pectoral nerve** (C8–T1) curves forwards between the axillary artery and vein to unite with a branch from the lateral pectoral nerve before entering the deep surface of the pectoralis minor muscle which they both supply.
2. The **medial cutaneous nerve of the arm** (C8–T1) is distributed to the skin on the medial aspect of the arm but also extends onto the anterior and posterior aspects of the distal third of the arm.
3. The **medial cutaneous nerve of the forearm** (C8–T1) is distributed to the skin on the medial side of the forearm as far distally as the wrist, via anterior and posterior branches.

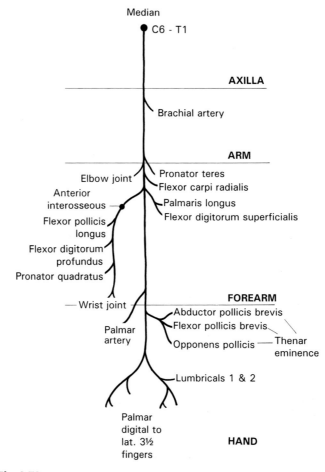

Fig. 3.72
The distribution of the median nerve.

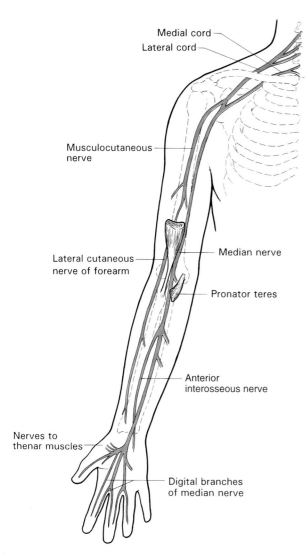

Fig. 3.73
The course and distribution of the median and musculocutaneous nerves.

articular branches to the elbow, wrist, intercarpal, carpometacarpal and intermetacarpal joints. In the forearm it supplies the flexor carpi ulnaris muscle and the medial half of the flexor digitorum profundus. Within the hand, it supplies the palmaris brevis muscle, the 3 short muscles of the hypothenar eminence, adductor pollicis, the third and fourth lumbricals and all the interossei. It is also responsible for the cutaneous supply to the palm of the hand via the palmar cutaneous branch and the palmar aspect of the medial $1\frac{1}{2}$ fingers as well as their dorsal aspect as far proximally as the base of the distal phalanx.

5. Anterior to the axillary artery, the medial root of the **median nerve** (C8–T1) unites with the lateral root from the lateral cord to form the median nerve (C6–T1). It descends into the arm lateral to the brachial artery and at the level of the coracobrachialis muscle adopts a position anterior to the artery before descending to the medial aspect of the cubital fossa (Fig. 3.73). Here it lies in front of the brachialis muscle but behind the bicipital aponeurosis. The median nerve enters the forearm between the 2 heads of the pronator teres muscle, crossing from the medial to the lateral side of the ulnar artery. It then descends through the forearm deep to the flexor digitorum superficialis muscle and superficial to the flexor digitorum profundus muscle. It becomes superficial at the wrist as it emerges at the lateral edge of the superficial flexor, proximal to the flexor retinaculum. It then gains access to the hand by passing deep to the flexor retinaculum through the carpal tunnel. Once in the hand it divides into a variable number of terminal branches. During its course through the arm, the medial nerve gives off vascular branches to the brachial artery and the nerve to the pronator teres muscle usually arises from above the elbow joint. In the forearm, the median nerve gives articular branches to the elbow joint and muscular branches to the flexor carpi radialis, palmaris longus (if present) and flexor digitorum superficialis. The remaining muscular branches arise from the anterior interosseous branch of the median nerve, which arises from the posterior aspect of the median nerve as it passes between the two heads of the pronator teres muscle. Accompanied by the anterior interosseous artery (a branch of the ulnar artery) the nerve passes distally on the interosseous membrane that connects the radius and ulna. Throughout its course, the anterior interosseous nerve supplies the flexor pollicis longus, the lateral half of the flexor digitorum profundus and the pronator quadratus muscles before terminating in articular branches that supply the wrist and intercarpal joints.

A palmar cutaneous branch arises proximal to the flexor retinaculum and supplies the skin over the region of the thenar eminence. In the hand, the

4. The **ulnar nerve** (C8–T1) runs distally through the axilla, medial to the axillary artery and the brachial artery, until the middle of the arm (Fig. 3.74). It then pierces the medial intermuscular septum and descends to the interval between the medial epicondyle of the humerus and the olecranon process of the ulna. It then enters the forearm between the two heads of the flexor carpi ulnaris muscle and descends along the medial side of the forearm lying on the flexor digitorum profundus muscle (Fig. 3.75). In the lower two-thirds of the forearm the nerve lies medial to the ulnar artery. It then passes into the hand superficial to the flexor retinaculum, lateral to the pisiform and medial to the ulnar artery before terminating into superficial and deep branches. Its course throughout the forearm is represented by a line drawn from the medial epicondyle to the lateral edge of the pisiform. Throughout its course it supplies

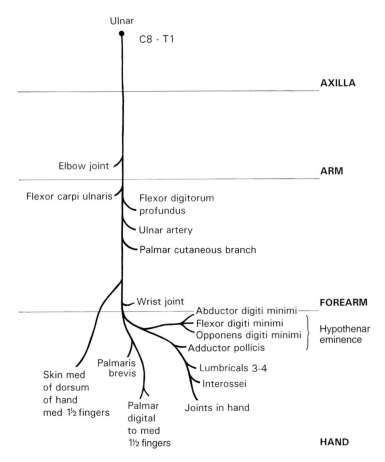

Ulnar
C8 - T1

AXILLA

Elbow joint

ARM

Flexor carpi ulnaris

Flexor digitorum profundus

Ulnar artery

Palmar cutaneous branch

Wrist joint

FOREARM

Abductor digiti minimi
Flexor digiti minimi
Opponens digiti minimi } Hypothenar eminence
Adductor pollicis

Palmaris brevis

Lumbricals 3-4

Interossei

Skin med of dorsum of hand med 1½ fingers

Palmar digital to med 1½ fingers

Joints in hand

HAND

Fig. 3.74
The distribution of the ulnar nerve.

median nerve supplies muscular branches to the 3 small muscles of the thenar eminence and the first and second lumbricals. The remaining branches of the median nerve supply the joints and skin of the lateral $3\frac{1}{2}$ fingers, including the dorsal aspect of these digits, as far proximally as the base of the distal phalanges.

Posterior cord
There are 5 terminal branches from the posterior cord of the brachial plexus, which is formed from the posterior divisions of the 3 trunks and carries fibers from the C5–T1 ventral rami of the spinal nerves:

1. The **upper subscapular nerve** (C5–C6) supplies the cranial part of the subscapularis muscle.
2. The **lower subscapular nerve** (C5–C6) is the larger of the two subscapular branches and supplies the caudal portion of the subscapularis muscle, terminating in the teres major muscle.
3. The **thoracodorsal nerve** (C6–C8) arises from the posterior cord between the 2 subscapular nerves. It accompanies the subscapular artery along the posterior wall of the axilla and supplies the latissimus dorsi muscle.
4. The **axillary nerve** (C5–C6) initially lies posterior to

the axillary artery and in front of the subscapularis muscle (Fig. 3.76). At the lower border of that muscle it winds backwards with the posterior circumflex humeral vessels and passes through the quadrangular space to supply branches to the shoulder joint before terminating in anterior and posterior divisions. The anterior branch continues along its course with the posterior circumflex humeral vessels and winds around the surgical neck of the humerus deep to the deltoid muscle which it supplies. It also sends some small cutaneous perforating branches to the skin over the lower regions of deltoid. The posterior division supplies the teres minor muscle and the posterior fibers of deltoid. The nerve appears at the lower border of deltoid and continues as the upper lateral cutaneous nerve of the arm.

5. The **radial nerve** (C5–T1) is the largest terminal branch of the brachial plexus and descends behind the axillary artery and upper part of the brachial artery in front of the subscapularis muscle (Fig. 3.77). It passes with the profunda brachii artery between the long and medial heads of the triceps muscle. It then passes obliquely in the spiral groove on the humerus to reach the lateral side of the bone,

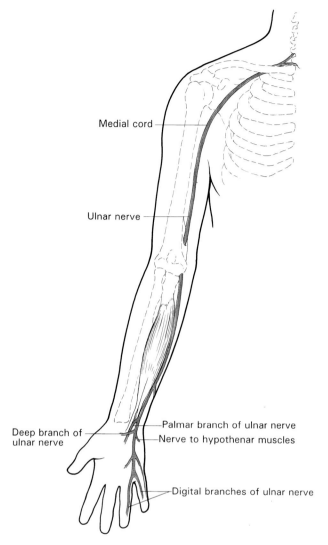

Fig. 3.75
The course and distribution of the ulnar nerve.

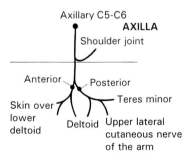

Fig. 3.76
The distribution of the axillary nerve.

where it pierces the lateral intermuscular septum to enter the anterior compartment of the arm (Fig. 3.78). It descends between the brachialis and the brachioradialis to reach the front of the lateral

epicondyle where it terminates in superficial and deep branches. Whilst in the axilla, the radial nerve gives off the posterior cutaneous nerve of the arm which supplies the skin on the dorsal surface as far inferiorly as the olecranon process. The muscular branches supply the triceps, anconeus, brachioradialis, extensor carpi radialis longus muscles and a small part of the brachialis muscle. During its course through the arm, the radial nerve gives rise to the lower lateral cutaneous nerve of the arm and the posterior cutaneous nerve of the forearm as well as sending branches to the elbow joint.

The superficial terminal branch of the radial nerve descends along the front of the lateral side of the upper two-thirds of the forearm, lying at first on the supinator and lateral to the radial artery. In the middle third of the forearm it lies behind the brachioradialis lying

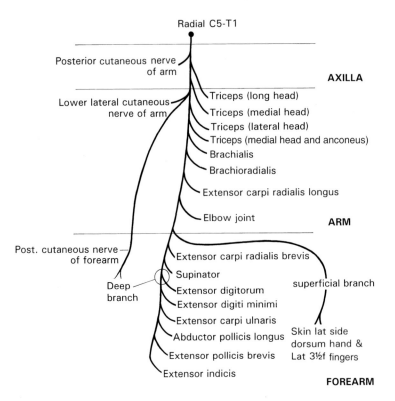

Fig. 3.77
The distribution of the radial nerve.

firstly on the pronator teres and then on the flexor digitorum superficialis and then on the flexor pollicis longus. At the wrist it passes deep to the tendon of the brachioradialis before dividing into 5 dorsal digital nerves which supply the skin on the radial side of the thumb and thenar eminence and the dorsal surface of the lateral $3\frac{1}{2}$ fingers as far distally as the base of the distal phalanx. The deep terminal branch of the radial nerve winds around the lateral side of the radius and descends on the posterior surface of the interosseous membrane. In its course through the forearm it supplies muscular branches to the extensor carpi radialis brevis, supinator, extensor digitorum, extensor digiti minimi, extensor carpi ulnaris, abductor pollicis longus, extensor pollicis longus, extensor pollicis brevis and extensor indicis. Articular branches are distributed to the carpal, distal radio-ulnar, intercarpal, intermetacarpal, metacarpophalangeal and proximal interphalangeal joints.

Ventral rami of the thoracic nerves

There are 12 pairs of thoracic spinal nerves and they exit from the vertebral column below the vertebra of the corresponding number. The upper 11 thoracic nerves pass anteriorly between the ribs and are termed intercostal nerves, whilst the 12th (subcostal) passes below the last rib. The presence of ribs ensures that there is no thoracic plexus. The nerves distribute sensory and motor information to and from the lateral and anterior surfaces of the thoracic and abdominal walls (Fig. 3.79). Each nerve is connected to an appropriate ganglion on the sympathetic chain by gray and white rami communicantes.

Shortly after exiting from the intervertebral foramen, the ventral ramus of the T1 nerve terminates in a large branch which passes into the brachial plexus and a small branch which forms the first intercostal nerve. The ventral rami of T2–T6 pass forward in the appropriate intercostal spaces occupying a position below the intercostal vessels. Posteriorly, the nerves pass between the pleura (supplying the parietal pleura) and the posterior intercostal membrane and as they run forwards they pass between the internal intercostal muscle and the subcostal muscles (Fig. 3.79). Throughout their course they supply both muscular branches to the intercostal muscles, the serratus posterior and the transverse thoracis muscles, and lateral and anterior cutaneous branches that supply the skin over the lateral and anterior aspects of the thoracic wall respectively. The lateral cutaneous branch of T2, the intercostobrachial nerve, communicates with the

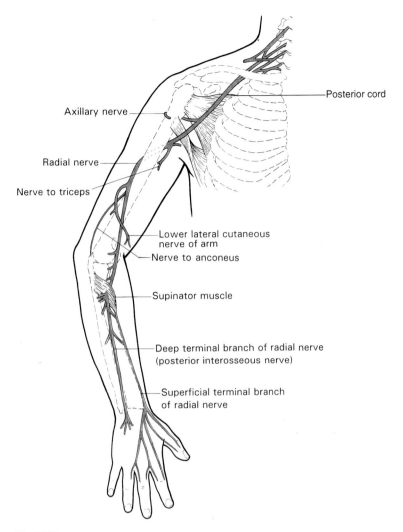

Posterior cord

Axillary nerve

Radial nerve

Nerve to triceps

Lower lateral cutaneous
nerve of arm

Nerve to anconeus

Supinator muscle

Deep terminal branch of radial nerve
(posterior interosseous nerve)

Superficial terminal branch
of radial nerve

Fig. 3.78
The course and distribution of the axillary and radial nerves.

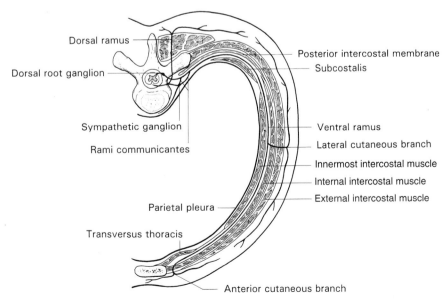

Dorsal ramus

Dorsal root ganglion

Sympathetic ganglion

Rami communicantes

Posterior intercostal membrane

Subcostalis

Ventral ramus

Lateral cutaneous branch

Innermost intercostal muscle

Internal intercostal muscle

External intercostal muscle

Parietal pleura

Transversus thoracis

Anterior cutaneous branch

Fig. 3.79
The course and distribution of a typical thoracic nerve.

medial cutaneous nerve of the arm and so has a distribution in the upper limb. The ventral rami of T7–T11 pass in a similar course to the upper intercostal nerves, but due to the lateral disposition of the lower thoracic wall, they also pass forwards into the anterior abdominal wall. Here, they supply rectus abdominis, external oblique, internal oblique and transversus abdominis muscles and carry sensory information from the diaphragm.

The subcostal nerve (T12) is larger than any of the other thoracic nerves and passes along the lower border of the 12th rib to gain access to the anterior abdominal wall. In addition to supplying the same structures as the other thoracic nerves, it supplies the skin over the anterior aspect of the gluteal region.

Lumbar plexus

The lumbar plexus is formed from the ventral rami of L1–L3 with some contribution from the L4 level (Fig. 3.80). It is formed within the substance of the psoas major muscle, anterior to the transverse processes of the lumbar vertebrae (Fig. 3.81). L1 receives a small twig from T12 and then splits into upper and lower branches. The upper branch bifurcates into the iliohypogastric and ilioinguinal nerves whereas the lower branch unites with a twig from L2 to form the genitofemoral nerve. The remainder of L2 and all of L3 and L4 divide into ventral and dorsal branches. The ventral branch of L2 unites with those of L3 and L4 to form the obturator nerve. The dorsal branches of L2 and L3 divide into smaller branches which unite to form the lateral cutaneous nerve of the thigh and larger branches which unite with the dorsal branch of L4 to form the femoral nerve. An accessory obturator nerve may arise from the ventral branches of L3 and L4. The lumbosacral trunk (L4–L5) contributes to the formation of the lumbosacral plexus (see below).

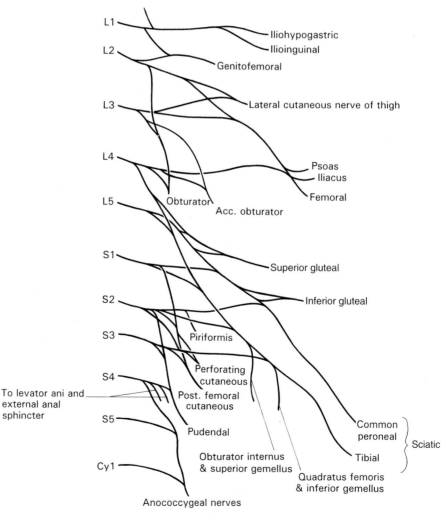

Fig. 3.80
The lumbosacral plexus.

> ### TERMINAL BRANCHES OF THE LUMBAR PLEXUS
>
> *Muscular*   quadratus lumborum (T12–L3)   psoas minor (L1)
>   psoas major (L2–L4)   iliacus (L2–L3)
>
> iliohypogastric (L1), ilioinguinal (L1), genitofemoral (L1–L2),
> lateral cutaneous nerve of the thigh (L2–L3), femoral (L2–L4),
> obturator (L2–L4)   accessory obturator (L3–L4).

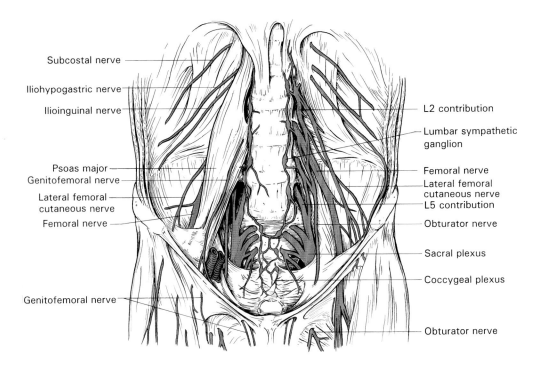

Fig. 3.81
The lumbosacral plexus.

The **iliohypogastric nerve** emerges from the lateral border of the psoas major muscle and passes obliquely across the quadratus lumborum muscle behind the lower pole of the kidney. It perforates the transversus abdominis muscle just above the iliac crest and divides into anterior and lateral cutaneous branches. The former runs between the internal oblique and transversus abdominis muscles, and supples both before piercing the external oblique approximately 3 cm above the superficial inguinal ring. The anterior cutaneous branch is distributed to the skin over the anterior aspect of the abdomen above the pubis. The lateral cutaneous branch pierces the external oblique to supply the skin over the posterolateral aspect of the gluteal region.

The **ilioinguinal nerve** emerges at the lateral border

of the psoas major muscle just caudal to the iliohypogastric nerve with which it communicates. It passes obliquely across the quadratus lumborum before perforating the transversus abdominis muscle at the anterior aspect of the iliac crest. It then pierces the internal oblique, which it supplies, and accompanies the spermatic cord/round ligament of the uterus through the superficial inguinal ring. In the male it is distributed to the skin over the superiomedial aspect of the thigh, the root of the penis and the upper part of the scrotum. In the female it supplies a corresponding region of skin in the thigh and the skin of the mons pubis and adjacent areas of the labia majora.

The **genitofemoral nerve** passes through the psoas major and emerges on its anterior aspect opposite the third and fourth lumbar vertebrae. It descends on this

138

muscle, deep to the peritoneum and passes behind the ureter before dividing into genital and femoral branches superior to the inguinal ligament. The genital branch passes through the inguinal canal via the deep inguinal ring to supply the cremaster muscle and skin of the scrotum in the male and the skin of the mons pubis and labia majora in the female. The femoral branch descends lateral to the external iliac artery and then deep to the circumflex iliac artery to enter the femoral sheath lateral to the femoral artery. It supplies the skin over the upper part of the femoral triangle.

The **lateral cutaneous nerve of the thigh** appears at the lateral border of the psoas major and obliquely crosses the iliacus as it passes towards the anterior superior iliac spine. Throughout its course it supplies branches to the parietal peritoneum. On the right side it passes behind and lateral to the caecum and on the left it passes behind the descending colon. It then passes behind the inguinal ligament before entering the thigh. It terminates in anterior and posterior branches with the former supplying the skin over the anterior and lateral aspects of the thigh as far inferiorly as the knee, and the latter supply the skin over the lateral aspect of the thigh from the greater trochanter to the mid-region of the thigh.

The **obturator nerve** descends through the psoas major muscle and at the pelvic inlet it runs behind the common iliac vessels and passes down and forwards along the lateral wall of the pelvis lying on the obturator internus muscle (Fig. 3.82). It passes through the obturator foramen to gain entry to the thigh, where it terminates in anterior and posterior branches. The

anterior branch exits from the pelvis and passes in front of the adductor brevis muscle and deep to the pectineus and adductor longus muscles to take part in the formation of the subsartorial plexus. As well as supplying the adductors brevis and longus, pectineus and gracilis muscles, the nerve supplies the skin over the medial aspect of the thigh and the hip joint, and sends vascular branches to the femoral artery (Fig. 3.83). The posterior branch pierces the obturator externus muscle, which it supplies, and passes deep to the adductor brevis and superficial to the medial part of the adductor magnus muscle which it also supplies. In addition, the posterior branch gives rise to articular branches which supply the knee joint and vascular branches which supply the popliteal artery.

The **femoral nerve** is the largest terminal branch of the lumbar plexus (Fig. 3.84). It descends through the psoas major muscle and emerges at its lateral border passing superficial to the iliacus muscle (Fig. 3.85). It supplies branches to the iliacus and gives rise to the nerve to the pectineus muscle. The femoral nerve then passes behind the inguinal ligament to enter the thigh lateral to the femoral artery where it terminates in anterior and posterior branches. The anterior branch gives rise to the intermediate and medial cutaneous nerves of the thigh and the posterior branch gives rise to the saphenous nerve and muscular branches to the quadriceps femoris muscle. The **saphenous nerve** is the largest cutaneous branch of the femoral nerve and descends lateral to the femoral artery to enter the adductor canal where it passes in front of the artery. It then descends vertically down the medial aspect of the

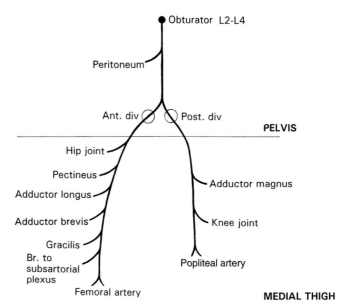

Fig. 3.82
The distribution of the obturator nerve.

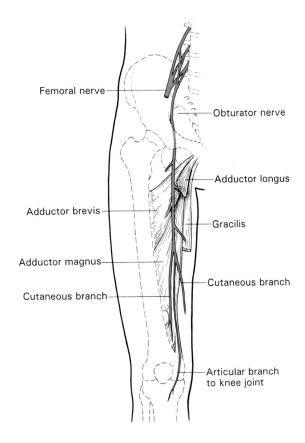

Fig. 3.83
The course and distribution of the obturator nerve.

Figure labels: Femoral nerve, Obturator nerve, Adductor longus, Adductor brevis, Gracilis, Adductor magnus, Cutaneous branch, Cutaneous branch, Articular branch to knee joint

knee and continues down the medial side of the leg with the long saphenous vein, supplying the skin of the medial aspect of the leg throughout its course. Some branches terminate at the level of the ankle joint, whereas others pass in front of the ankle joint and supply the skin on the medial side of the foot, often as far as the first metatarsophalangeal joint. The femoral nerve supplies vascular branches to the femoral artery and articular branches to the hip, knee and ankle joints.

Sacral plexus

The sacral plexus is formed from the lumbosacral trunk (L4–L5) and the ventral rami of S1–S4 (Fig. 3.80). The plexus is located on the posterior wall of the pelvis anterior to the piriformis muscle but deep to the internal iliac vessels, the ureter and the sigmoid colon on the left, and the terminal coils of the ileum on the right. Each of the spinal nerves from L4 to S3 terminates in ventral and dorsal divisions.

SACRAL PLEXUS

Branches from ventral divisions

Nerve to quadratus femoris and inferior gemellus (L4–S1)
Nerve to obturator internus and superior gemellus (L5–S2)
Posterior femoral cutaneous (S2–S3)
Tibial (L4–S3)
Pudendal (S2–S4)

Branches from dorsal divisions

Nerve to piriformis (S2)
Superior gluteal (L4–S1)
Inferior gluteal (L5–S2)
Posterior femoral cutaneous (S1–S2)
Common peroneal (L4–S2)
Perforating cutaneous (S2–S3)

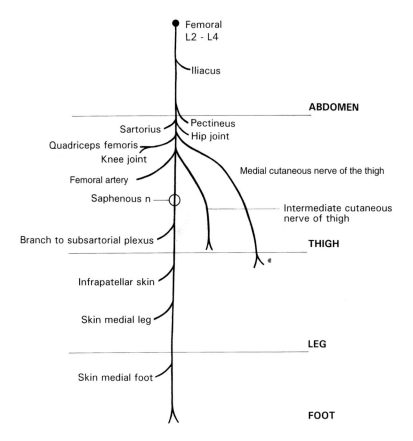

Fig. 3.84
The distribution of the femoral nerve.

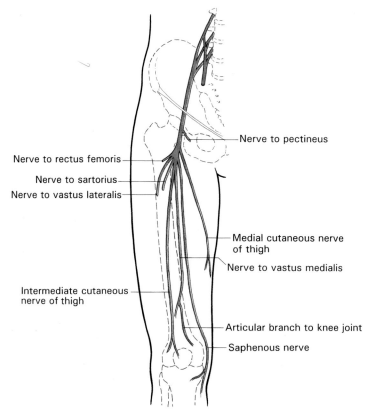

Fig. 3.85
The course and distribution of the femoral nerve.

The **nerve to the quadratus femoris and the inferior gemellus** exits from the pelvis via the greater sciatic foramen under cover of the piriformis muscle. It descends on the ischium, deep to the sciatic nerve, to supply the two named muscles and an articular branch to the hip joint.

The **nerve to the obturator internus and the superior gemellus** also exits from the pelvis via the greater sciatic foramen under cover of the piriformis. It supplies a branch to the superior gemellus muscle and then passes over the ischial spine, lateral to the internal pudendal vessels, before re-entering the pelvis via the lesser sciatic foramen to supply the obturator internus muscle.

The **nerve to the piriformis** is derived from the dorsal division of the S2 nerve as it exits from the anterior sacral foramen. It then passes directly into the anterior surface of the muscle.

The **superior gluteal nerve** exits from the pelvis into the gluteal region via the greater sciatic foramen. It passes above the piriformis muscle and is accompanied by the superior gluteal vessels. It terminates by dividing into superior and inferior branches. The former perforate and supply the gluteus medius muscle and the latter supply the gluteus medius, gluteus minimus and the tensor fasciae latae.

The **inferior gluteal nerve** also exits via the greater sciatic foramen but below the piriformis muscle and is accompanied by the inferior gluteal vessels. It supplies the gluteus maximus muscle.

The **posterior femoral cutaneous nerve** exits via the greater sciatic foramen below the piriformis and descends under cover of the gluteus maximus muscle in company with the inferior gluteal artery. It passes through the posterior fascial compartment of the thigh superficial to the long head of biceps femoris and deep to the fasciae latae before piercing the deep fascia at the back of the knee. In the leg it accompanies the short saphenous vein as far as midway down the calf. Throughout its course it gives off gluteal and perineal branches with terminal branches to the thigh and leg. The gluteal nerves are 3 or 4 in number and supply the skin over the lower lateral part of the gluteus maximus muscle. The perineal branches supply the skin over the upper medial aspect of the thigh and pass to the scrotum in the male and the labia majora in the female. The branches in the thigh and leg are numerous and supply the skin over the back and medial aspects of the thigh, popliteal fossa and upper aspect of the back of the calf.

The **perforating cutaneous nerve** pierces the sacrotuberous ligament to supply the skin over the medial and lower aspects of the skin covering the gluteus maximus.

The **pudendal nerve** leaves the pelvis via the greater sciatic foramen below the piriformis and superficial to the coccygeus muscle (Fig. 3.86). It crosses the sacrospinous

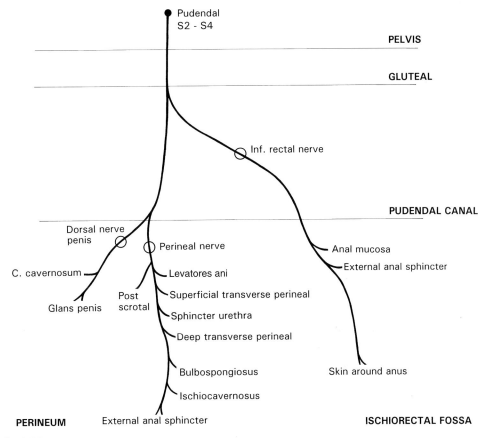

Fig. 3.86
The distribution of the pudendal nerve.

ligament medial to the internal pudendal vessels and accompanies the internal pudendal artery through the lesser sciatic foramen, where it passes into the pudendal canal on the lateral wall of the ischiorectal fossa (Fig. 3.87). In the canal it gives off the inferior rectal nerve and divides into the perineal nerve and the dorsal nerve of the penis/clitoris. The **inferior rectal nerve** pierces the medial wall of the pudendal canal and crosses the ischiorectal fossa in company with the internal rectal vessels. It is distributed to the external anal sphincter, the mucosal lining of the lower part of the anal canal and the skin around the anus. The **perineal nerve** passes through the pudendal canal below the internal pudendal artery and accompanies the perineal artery before terminating in the posterior scrotal/labial and muscular branches. The medial and lateral posterior scrotal/labial nerves supply the skin of the scrotum and the labia majora. The muscular branches are distributed to the superficial and deep transverse perineal muscles, the bulbospongiosus and ischiocavernosus muscles, the sphincter urethrae and the anterior parts of the external anal sphincter and levator ani. The **dorsal nerve of the penis/clitoris** also passes through the pudendal canal but above the internal pudendal artery along the ischial ramus. It sends a branch to the corpus cavernosum and runs with the dorsal artery of the penis/clitoris to end in the glans penis/clitoris.

The **sciatic nerve** is formed from the union of the **tibial** and **common peroneal** nerves of the sacral plexus (Fig. 3.88). This is the largest nerve in the body and it exist from the pelvis via the greater sciatic foramen, deep to the piriformis. In the gluteal region it descends under cover of the gluteus maximus muscle between the greater trochanter of the femur and the ischial tuberosity. As it descends it lies on the ischium and then crosses the obturator internus and gemelli muscles before passing over the quadratus femoris. It is accompanied on its medial side by the posterior cutaneous nerve of the thigh and the inferior gluteal artery and descends through the posterior fascial compartment of the thigh on the adductor magnus muscle. At a variable location in the thigh the sciatic nerve will split into its original components of the tibial nerve formed from the ventral divisions of the L4–S3 spinal nerves and the common peroneal nerve formed from the dorsal divisions of the L4–S2 spinal nerves. The sciatic nerve gives articular branches to the hip joint and muscular branches to the hamstring muscles, i.e. biceps femoris, semimembranosus, semitendinosus and the ischial head of adductor magnus.

The **tibial nerve** is the larger of the 2 terminal branches of the sciatic nerve (Fig. 3.89) and descends through the posterior fascial compartment of the thigh to reach the popliteal fossa where it lies lateral to the popliteal vessels (Fig. 3.90). It then passes deep to the soleus muscle and continues into the leg where it descends with the posterior tibial vessels to occupy a position between the calcaneus and the medial malleolus. It passes deep to the flexor retinaculum and terminates in the medial and lateral plantar nerves. Throughout its course, the tibial nerve gives rise to a number of branches. Articular branches supply the knee and ankle joints, vascular twigs supply the accompanying vessels and muscular branches supply the gastrocnemius, plantaris, soleus, popliteus, tibialis posterior, flexor digitorum longus and flexor hallucis longus. The **sural nerve** arises between the 2 heads of the gastrocnemius muscle and is joined by the sural communicating branch from the common peroneal

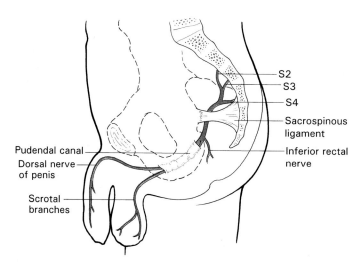

Fig. 3.87
The course and distribution of the pudendal nerve.

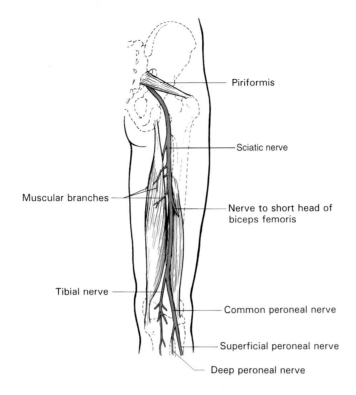

Piriformis

Sciatic nerve

Muscular branches

Nerve to short head of biceps femoris

Tibial nerve

Common peroneal nerve

Superficial peroneal nerve

Deep peroneal nerve

Fig. 3.88
The course and distribution of the sciatic nerve.

nerve. It then descends along the lateral border of the tendo calcaneus to occupy a position between the calcaneus and the lateral malleolus. It is responsible for the cutaneous supply to the lateral and posterior aspects of the lower third of the leg and the lateral side of the foot. A medial calcaneal branch is also given off which supplies the skin over the heel and the medial side of the sole of the foot.

The **medial plantar nerve** is the larger of the 2 terminal divisions and it passes in company with the medial plantar artery. Its course runs deep to the abductor hallucis muscle where it gives rise to a digital branch which supplies the skin of the medial side of the large toe. The medial plantar nerve gives rise to a number of articular, muscular and cutaneous nerves. Articular branches supply the appropriate tarsal and metatarsal joints in this region; muscular branches supply the abductor hallucis, flexor digitorum brevis, flexor hallucis brevis and first lumbrical muscles; and cutaneous branches pass into the medial aspect of the sole of the foot. The medial plantar nerve then divides into 3 common plantar digital nerves at the base of the metatarsals and these pass between the divisions of the plantar aponeurosis before splitting into 2 proper digital nerves. The first supplies the skin of the adjacent sides of the great and second toes; the second supplies contiguous sides of the second and third toes; and the third supplies adjacent surfaces of the third and fourth

toes. In addition, each proper digital nerve supplies articular branches to immediate joints, and fibers pass onto the dorsal aspect of the toes to supply the appropriate nail beds.

The **lateral plantar nerve** passes with the lateral plantar artery towards the tubercle of the fifth metatarsal. Along its course it supplies branches to the flexor accessorius and abductor digit minimi muscles as well as cutaneous branches to the lateral aspect of the sole of the foot. The nerve then bifurcates into superficial and deep branches. The superficial branch bifurcates almost immediately into 2 plantar digital nerves, the lateral of which supplies the skin over the lateral aspect of the fifth toe, the flexor digiti minimi brevis muscle and the interossei of the fourth space, whilst the medial branch supplies the skin on contiguous sides of the fourth and fifth toes. The deep branch of the lateral plantar nerve supplies the second, third and fourth lumbricals, the adductor hallucis, and all the remaining interossei.

The **common peroneal nerve** descends obliquely to the lateral side of the popliteal fossa and the fibular head (Fig. 3.91). The upper part of this nerve gives rise to the lateral cutaneous nerve of the calf which supplies the skin over the anterior, posterior and lateral aspects of the proximal calf and articular branches to the knee and the superior tibiofibular joint. It also gives rise to the **sural communicating nerve** which will ultimately

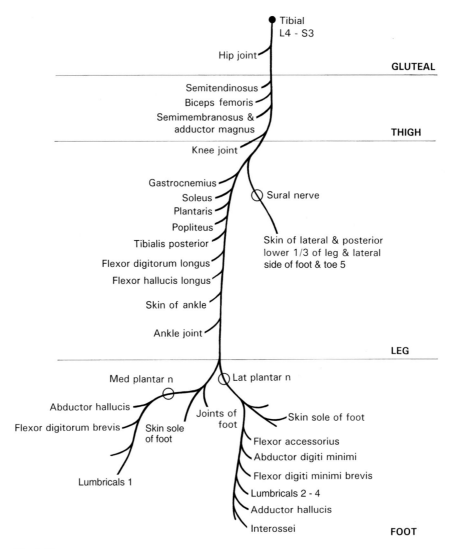

Fig. 3.89
The distribution of the tibial nerve.

join with the sural branch of the tibial nerve. As the common peroneal nerve winds around the lateral aspect of the neck of the fibula it bifurcates into superficial and deep branches within the substance of the peroneus longus muscle (Fig. 3.92). The **superficial peroneal nerve** passes between the peroneal muscles and the extensor digitorum longus giving off branches to both the peroneus longus and brevis and the skin over the lower part of the leg. It then terminates in medial and lateral branches, with the former passing in front of the ankle joint to bifurcate into 2 dorsal digital nerves which supply the medial aspect of the large toe and the skin on the adjacent surfaces of the second and third toes. The lateral branch also terminates in dorsal digital branches, which supply contiguous surfaces of the third and fourth, and fourth and fifth toes as well as the skin over the lateral aspect of the ankle. The **deep peroneal** branch of the common peroneal nerve (also

known as the anterior tibial nerve) passes deep to the extensor digitorum longus to reach the anterior aspect of the interosseous membrane, which it descends in company with the anterior tibial artery. Throughout its course in the leg it sends articular branches to the ankle and muscular branches to the tibialis anterior, extensor hallucis longus, extensor digitorum longus and peroneus tertius muscles. The nerve passes anterior to the ankle joint and bifurcates into lateral and medial branches. The lateral branch supplies the extensor digitorum brevis muscle, tarsal joints and the metatarsophalangeal joints of toes two to four. The medial branch passes lateral to the dorsalis pedis artery to the first interosseous space and terminates in 2 dorsal digital nerves which supply adjacent surfaces of the great and second toes and the first dorsal interosseous muscle.

The **pelvic splanchnic nerves** are visceral branches

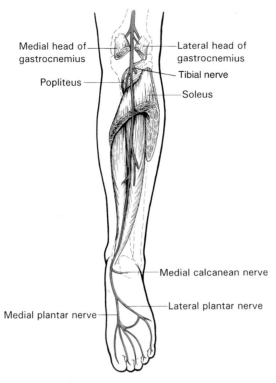

Fig. 3.90
The course and distribution of the tibial nerve.

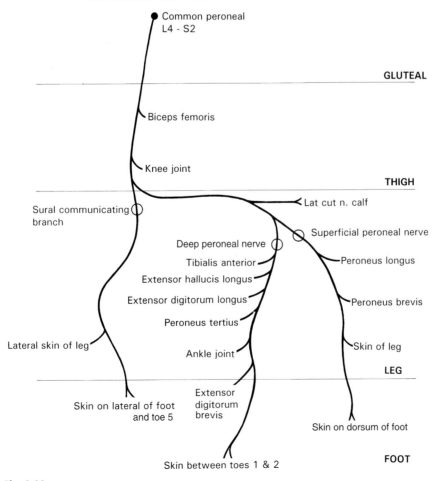

Fig. 3.91
The distribution of the common peroneal nerve.

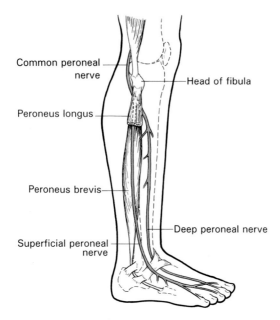

Fig. 3.92
The course and distribution of the common peroneal nerve.

arise from the ventral rami of S2–S4 and will be considered with the section on the autonomic nervous system (p. 154). In addition, muscular branches arise from the S4 nerve and supply the levator ani and coccygeus muscles and the external anal sphincter.

The **coccygeal plexus** is small and forms a loop involving a descending branch from S4 with the ventral ramus of S5 and C1. These anococcygeal nerves pierce the sacrotuberous ligament and supply the skin over the coccyx.

THE AUTONOMIC NERVOUS SYSTEM

The autonomic division of the nervous system acts to regulate the organs and structures concerned with digestion, circulation, respiration, excretion and the maintenance of body temperature by controlling visceral reflexes, smooth and cardiac muscle activity and glandular secretions. Although there are both sensory and motor components, the system is principally subdivided on the basis of its motor function into sympathetic and parasympathetic parts. The former system prepares the body for urgent

activity, whilst the latter relaxes the body and controls functions at a normal level. However, rather than displaying any real independent function, these two divisions operate in a delicate harmony to maintain homeostasis.

Little is known about the **afferent** components of the autonomic nervous system but they do convey the sensation of visceral distension (fullness or emptiness) and visceral pain. They also serve a specific physiological role in the carotid body and sinus by monitoring carbon dioxide levels and arterial pressure respectively.

The major component of the autonomic nervous system is its **efferent** or motor output and Figure 3.93 summarises the basic distribution of the two divisions. The autonomic motor fibers occur in a 2- neuron chain (pre and postganglionic fibers) with the cell body of the primary neuron located in the visceral efferent column of the brain or spinal cord and the cell body of the secondary neuron occurring in a ganglion outside the cerebrospinal axis. In the parasympathetic system the preganglionic fibers tend to be long whilst the postganglionic fibers are very short and in the sympathetic system it is the postganglionic fibers that tend to be longer. The autonomic ganglia fall into 3 topographical locations:

1. The **paravertebral ganglia** occur in a chain of 21–22 connected swellings that sit in the paravertebral gutters. These form the sympathetic chain or trunk that extends from the cervical region above to the coccyx below
2. The **prevertebral ganglia** occur in association with the major arteries of the gut – celiac, superior and inferior mesenteric, and it is through the branches of these arteries that the postganglionic fibers reach their target organ. These ganglia are also associated with the sympathetic division of the autonomic nervous system.
3. The **peripheral ganglia** belong to the parasympathetic system and lie in close proximity to the effector tissue, e.g. the gastrointestinal tract, bladder.

Autonomic plexuses occur in the thorax, abdomen and pelvis and these are generally formed from both nerve fibers and ganglia carrying both sympathetic and parasympathetic components.

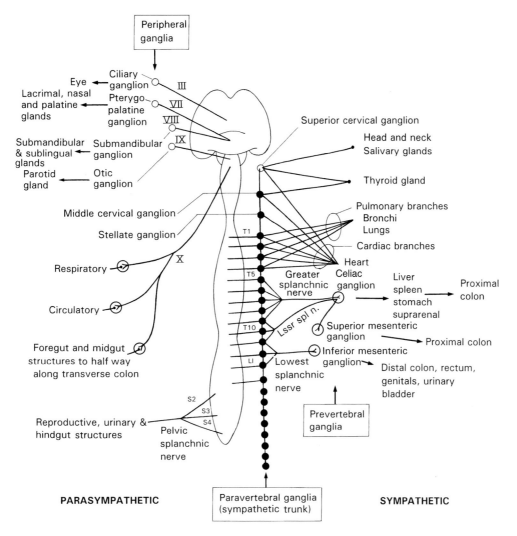

Fig. 3.93
Summary of the motor distribution of the autonomic nervous system.

SUMMARY OF AUTONOMIC FUNCTION

	Sympathetic	**Parasympathetic**
Blood vessels		
Skin	vasoconstriction	no innervation
Skeletal muscle	vasodilation	no innervation
Viscera (except heart and lungs)	vasoconstriction	no innervation
Iris	pupillary dilation	pupillary contraction
Ciliary muscle	no innervation	accommodation
Lacrimal, gastric, salivary, intestinal and pancreas glands	inhibitory	stimulates secretion
Sweat glands	sweat production	no innervation
Arrector pili muscles	contraction	no innervation
Heart	increases cardiac activity dilates coronary arteries	decreases cardiac activity constricts coronary arteries
Lungs	bronchodilatation	bronchoconstriction
Stomach and intestines	decreases motility	increases motility
Gall bladder	inhibits secretion	stimulates secretion
Suprarenal glands	stimulates secretion	no innervation
Bladder	relaxes muscle, contracts internal sphincter – urine retention	contracts muscle, relaxes internal sphincter – urine expulsion
Internal anal sphincter	contraction	relaxation

Visceral efferents

Sympathetic

The sympathetic system is the larger and more widely distributed division of the autonomic nervous system. It regulates functions that prepare the body for activity accompanied by an expenditure of energy by:
   a. increasing cardiac rate, blood pressure, blood sugar levels and respiratory activity
   b. dilating pupils,
   c. decreasing peristalsis
   d. decreasing the blood supply to the viscera and increasing the supply to the somatic muscles
   e. initiating smooth muscle contraction to the sphincters etc.

The efferents have a **thoracolumbar outflow** with the neurons originating in the intermediolateral cell column of spinal segments T1–L3. The axons of these preganglionic fibers exit from the spinal cord in the ventral roots of the spinal nerves T1–L3 and enter the sympathetic trunks via white rami communicantes. The paired sympathetic trunks are ganglionated cords that sit in the paravertebral gutters and extend from the base of the skull to the coccyx. The trunks lie anterior to the cervical transverse processes in the neck, anterior to the rib heads in the thorax, anterolateral to the lumbar vertebral bodies and medial to the anterior sacral foramina in the pelvis.

There are between 22 and 24 ganglia in each trunk – 3 cervical, usually 11 thoracic (although there may be 10 or 12), 4 lumbar and 4 sacral. Because of the restricted thoracolumbar outflow, it is only from these specific spinal nerves that white rami communicantes arise and pass into the sympathetic trunks. On entering the trunks the preganglionic fibers may follow 1 of 3 potential routes (Fig. 3.94):

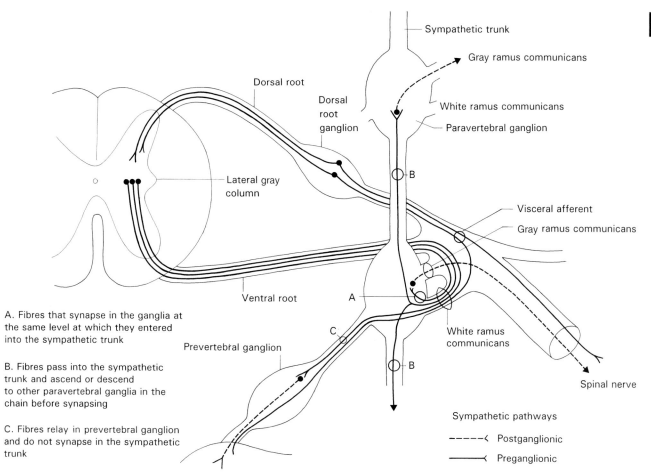

A. Fibres that synapse in the ganglia at the same level at which they entered into the sympathetic trunk

B. Fibres pass into the sympathetic trunk and either ascend or descend to other paravertebral ganglia in the chain before synapsing

C. Fibres relay in prevertebral ganglion and do not synapse in the sympathetic trunk

Fig. 3.94
The sympathetic motor pathways.

1. The preganglionic fibers can synapse in the ganglion near the spinal level at which they entered. From here the postganglionic fibers exit in the gray rami communicantes and enter the spinal nerve to supply the blood vessels, sweat glands and arrector pili muscles of the skin of the limbs and body wall. Fibers can also pass in plexuses to supply the thoracic viscera.

2. The preganglionic fibers may enter the sympathetic trunk and either descend or ascend within the trunk before synapsing in a ganglion at a different level. This occurs predominantly at the cranial and caudal poles of the trunk, where there are no white rami communicantes connecting directly to the upper and lower spinal nerves. Thus, autonomic fibers can only travel in these spinal nerves if they travel firstly in the sympathetic trunk. Once the fibers reach the appropriate ganglion in the sympathetic trunk, they will synapse with the postganglionic fibers and will then exit via the gray rami communicates to supply the skin and body wall and the thoracic viscera via the spinal nerves. The exception to this is the output from the superior cervical ganglion, which supplies the majority of the postganglionic sympathetic fibers for the head and neck.

3. to gain access to the abdominal and pelvic viscera, preganglionic fibers traverse the sympathetic trunk without synapsing and pass to the effector tissues via splanchnic nerves which terminate in 1 of 3 prevertebral ganglia. The postganglionic fibers pass into the plexuses that surround the main branches of the aorta and so are distributed with the arterial network.

Cervical part of the sympathetic trunk

There are 3 sympathetic ganglia in the cervical region – superior, middle and cervicothoracic (stellate). They receive no white rami communicantes but each sends a gray ramus communicantes to each of the cervical spinal nerves. The fibers originate in the upper thoracic segments of the spinal cord and ascend in the sympathetic trunk to reach the ganglia.

The **superior cervical ganglion** is the largest of the 3 ganglia and is found anterior to the transverse processes of C2 and C3. The **internal carotid nerve** arises from the superior pole of the ganglion and ascends around the internal carotid artery. In this way, the postganglionic fibers gain access to most tissues of the head and neck via a plexus around the various arterial branches.

Branches

1. Gray rami communicantes to C1–C4 spinal nerves.
2. Branches to the vagus and hypoglossal nerves.
3. Branches to the glossopharyngeal and vagus nerves to form the **jugular nerve** which ascends through the jugular foramen to supply the meninges of the posterior cranial fossa.
4. Laryngopharyngeal branches that supply the carotid body and pharynx and join with cranial nerves IX and X to form the pharyngeal plexus.
5. Cardiac branches which descend through the neck and into the thorax to be incorporated into the cardiac plexus.
6. Plexuses of postganglionic sympathetic fibers pass with the branches of the common carotid artery to supply much of the head and neck. Some fibers pass to parasympathetic peripheral ganglia but they will pass straight through without synapsing: (a) with the facial artery to reach the submandibular ganglion, (b) with the middle meningeal artery to reach the otic ganglion, (c) they condense to form the deep petrosal nerve which passes through the pterygoid canal with the greater petrosal nerve to

access the pterygopalatine ganglion, and (d) branches pass with the ophthalmic artery via the ciliary ganglion.

The **middle cervical ganglion** is the smallest of the cervical ganglia and is located medial to the carotid tubercle of C6 and anterior to the inferior thyroid artery (Fig. 3.95).

Branches

1. Gray rami communicantes to spinal nerves C5–C6.
2. Thyroid branches which travel with the inferior thyroid artery to both the thyroid and parathyroid glands.
3. Cardiac branches which form the largest branch of the cardiac plexus.
4. Anterior and posterior cords which connect it to the stellate ganglion. The posterior cord splits to enclose the vertebral artery and the anterior cord loops below and in front of the subclavian artery to form the **ansa subclavia**, which communicates with the phrenic nerve.
5. Branches to the trachea and esophagus.

The **stellate (cervicothoracic) ganglion** is larger than the middle ganglion and is probably formed from the union of the lower 2 cervical ganglia with the first thoracic ganglion. It is located anterior to, and between, the transverse process of C7 and the first rib, and posterior to the vertebral artery (Fig. 3.95).

Branches

1. Gray rami communicantes to spinal nerves C7–T1.
2. Cardiac branch which passes to the cardiac plexus.
3. Branches to blood vessels – these form extensive

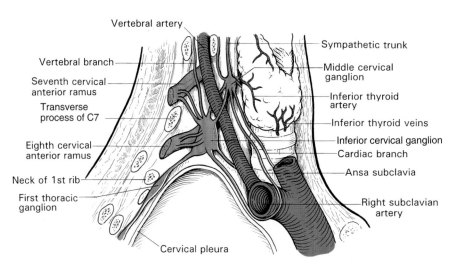

Fig. 3.95
The middle cervical and stellate sympathetic ganglia.

networks along the vertebral and subclavian arteries supplying postganglionic sympathetic fibers to the upper limb as far distally as the lower region of the axillary artery.

Thoracic ganglia

In general, the number of thoracic sympathetic ganglia corresponds with the number of thoracic spinal nerves, although the ganglion for T1 is often fused with the last cervical ganglion to form the stellate ganglion. The thoracic ganglia are located posterior to the costal pleura and anterior to the rib heads. The sympathetic trunk passes from the thorax into the abdomen posterior to the medial arcuate ligament of the diaphragm (Fig. 3.96).

Branches

1. White and gray rami communicantes to each of the thoracic spinal nerves.
2. Medial branches from the upper 5 ganglia give rise to vascular branches that pass to the aorta and are distributed with its branches.
3. Medial branches from ganglia 2–5 also pass to the posterior pulmonary and deep cardiac plexuses, from where small branches pass to the trachea and esophagus.
4. Medial branches from the lower 7 ganglia send branches to the aorta and unite to form the abdominal splanchnic nerves.

The **greater splanchnic nerve** consists mainly of preganglionic sympathetic fibers and visceral

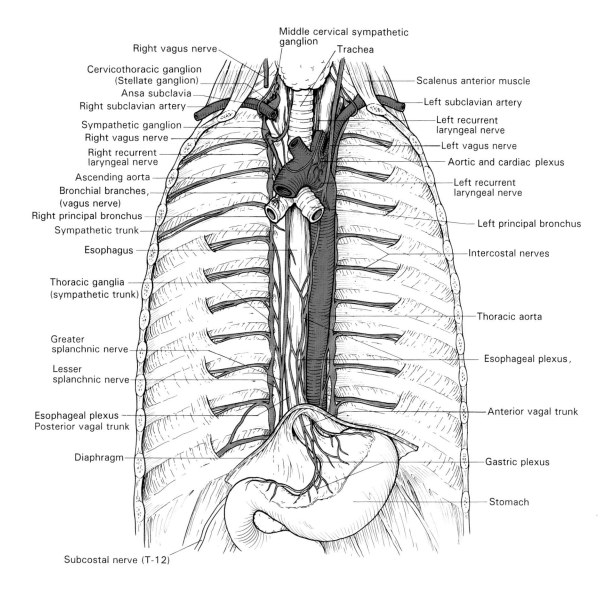

Fig. 3.96
The sympathetic trunks and vagus nerve in the thorax and upper abdomen.

afferents and is formed from the branches of thoracic ganglia 5–9 (and sometimes 10). The nerve descends on the vertebral bodies and sends branches to the aorta before perforating the crus of the diaphragm and terminating in the celiac prevertebral ganglion. From here, postganglionic fibers pass to the viscera of the foregut and midgut, i.e. stomach, liver, spleen, suprarenals, small gut, proximal colon etc.

The **lesser splanchnic nerve** is usually formed from branches of thoracic ganglia 9–10 and it enters the abdomen by piercing the diaphragm. The nerve may pass and relay through the celiac ganglion or it may pass directly to the superior mesenteric prevertebral ganglion. From here, postganglionic fibers generally pass to the region of the proximal colon.

The **lowest splanchnic nerve** is usually formed from the lowest thoracic and sometimes the upper 2 lumbar ganglia. It passes into the abdomen with the sympathetic trunk and terminates in the inferior mesenteric prevertebral ganglion. From here, postganglionic fibers pass to the distal colon, rectum, bladder, genitals, etc.

Lumbar ganglia

There are generally 4 or 5 lumbar ganglia and they are situated anterior to the vertebral column in the extraperitoneal connective tissue along the medial margin of the psoas major muscle. The lumbar ganglia lie posterior to the common iliac artery and are overlapped by the inferior vena cava on the right and the aortic lymph nodes on the left (Fig. 3.97).

Branches

1. White rami communicantes to L1, L2 and sometimes L3.

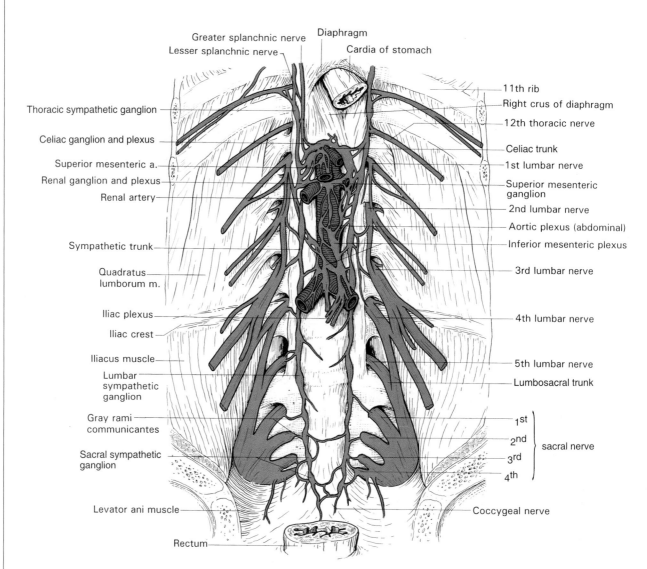

Fig. 3.97
The lumbar sympathetic trunk and abdominal autonomic ganglia.

2. Gray rami communicantes to L1–L5.
3. L1 and L2 may form part of the lowest splanchnic nerve.
4. Vascular branches to the aortic plexus and into the lower limbs as far as the proximal extent of the femoral artery.
5. Lumbar splanchnic nerves which pass down in front of the common iliac vessels to form the hypogastric plexuses.

Pelvic ganglia
The 4–5 pelvic ganglia lie in the extraperitoneal connective tissue of the pelvis, medial to the anterior sacral foramina.

Branches

1. Gray rami communicantes to the sacral and coccygeal spinal nerves.
2. Branches to the inferior hypogastric plexus.
3. Vascular branches to the popliteal artery (fibers originally travelled with the tibial nerve).

Parasympathetic

The parasympathetic efferents have a more localized effect than the sympathetic efferents and have a

craniosacral outflow. Parasympathetic efferent components are found in cranial nerves III, VII, IX and X and in sacral nerves 2–4. The cranial component is associated with 4 peripheral ganglia – ciliary, pterygopalatine, submandibular and otic, and the sacral component passes in the pelvic splanchnic nerves (Fig. 3.98).

Oculomotor nerve (III)
The parasympathetic efferents originate in the **accessory oculomotor nucleus** (Edinger–Westphal) of the midbrain. The preganglionic fibers travel with the third cranial nerve, which enters the orbit after traversing the cavernous sinus and the superior orbital fissure. The parasympathetic fibers travel in the branch to the inferior oblique muscle and terminate in the **ciliary ganglion**, which lies lateral to the ophthalmic artery between the optic nerve and the rectus lateralis muscle. The postganglionic fibers travel as **short ciliary nerves**, which pierce the sclera of the eye and supply the sphincter pupillae and ciliary muscle.

Facial nerve (VII)
The parasympathetic efferents originate in the **superior salivatory nucleus** of the pons. The preganglionic fibers pass with the nervus intermedius of the facial

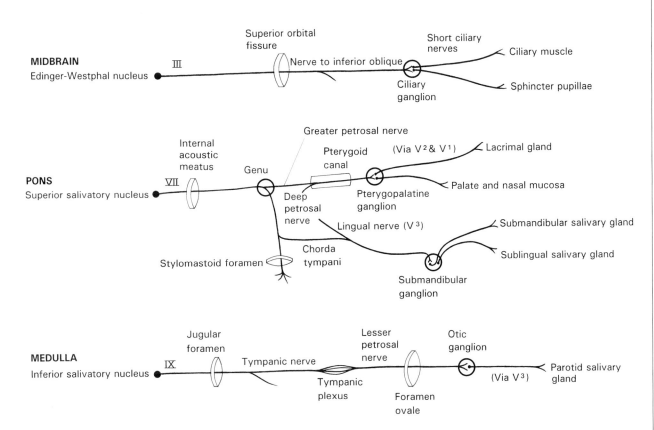

Fig. 3.98
Summary of the parasympathetic motor innervation of the head and neck.

nerve through the internal acoustic meatus to the inner ear. The **greater petrosal nerve** branches away at the genu and ascends into the middle cranial fossa before descending on its floor towards the foramen lacerum. At the opening to the pterygoid canal of the sphenoid bone, it is joined by the deep petrosal nerve (postganglionic sympathetic) to form the **nerve of the pterygoid canal**. The nerves pass into the pterygopalatine fossa and the parasympathetic fibers terminate in the **pterygopalatine ganglion**. The postganglionic parasympathetic fibers are secretomotor to the lacrimal gland and reach their destination by 'hitch-hiking' with the maxillary nerve, its zygomatic branch and then its zygomaticotemporal branch before reaching the gland via the lacrimal nerve (V[1]).

Other preganglionic parasympathetic fibers leave the facial nerve in its **chorda tympani** branch, which exits from the middle ear via the petrotympanic fissure. The chorda tympani joins the lingual nerve (V[3]) and fibers pass to the submandibular ganglion, which sits on the upper part of the hyoglossus muscle. From here, postganglionic fibers pass to the submandibular and sublingual salivary glands as secretomotor fibers.

Glossopharyngeal nerve (IX)
Parasympathetic efferent fibers originate in the **inferior salivatory nucleus** of the medulla and pass with the cranial nerve out through the jugular foramen. The parasympathetic fibers travel in its tympanic branch, which traverses the **tympanic plexus** and gives rise to the **lesser petrosal nerve**. This nerve ascends to the floor of the middle cranial fossa and descends to the foramen ovale through which it passes to terminate in the **otic ganglion**. Postganglionic fibers then pass with the auriculotemporal nerve (V[3]) to supply secretomotor fibers to the parotid salivary gland.

Vagus nerve (X)
The parasympathetic efferents in this cranial nerve have a wide distribution throughout the neck, thorax and abdomen to approximately halfway along the transverse colon (Fig. 3.93). The fibers arise in the **dorsal vagal nucleus** of the medulla and descend as pulmonary, cardiac, esophageal, gastric, intestinal and other branches. The function of these fibers is to slow the cardiac cycle, initiate bronchoconstriction, stimulate secretion of the gastric and intestinal glands and stimulate the muscular coat of the gut wall. The fibers relay in small ganglia which lie in the walls of the individual viscera, so that the postganglionic fibers are short compared to their preganglionic counterparts.

Pelvic splanchnic nerves (S2–S4)
Preganglionic parasympathetic efferents pass in the ventral roots of S2–S4 giving rise to the pelvic splanchnic nerves (Fig. 3.93). Again these fibers synapse with small ganglia in the walls of the viscera they supply, namely the rectum, bladder, penis/clitoris, testes/ovaries, uterine tubes and uterus. Fibers also pass upwards to supply the distal part of the transverse colon, the descending and sigmoid colon and the rectum.

Autonomic plexuses

The autonomic plexuses are an accumulation of nerves and ganglia in the trunk cavities that distribute fibers (both sympathetic and parasympathetic) to all the viscera via arterial branches. These plexuses (cardiac, pulmonary, celiac and hypogastric) give rise to a myriad of smaller named plexuses that adopt their name from the artery with which they are associated.

The **cardiac plexus** lies at the base of the heart and is topographically (but not functionally) separated into superficial and deep components. The **superficial (ventral) plexus** lies below the arch of the aorta, anterior to the right pulmonary artery. Its sympathetic component arises from the superior cervical ganglion of the sympathetic trunk as cardiac branches. Its parasympathetic component arises from the left vagus as 2 cervical cardiac branches. The superficial cardiac plexus, in turn, gives rise to connections to the deep cardiac plexus and the right coronary and left pulmonary plexuses. The **deep (dorsal) plexus** lies anterior to the bifurcation of the trachea above the division of the pulmonary trunk and posterior to the aortic arch. In addition to branches from the superficial plexus, its sympathetic component arises from cardiac branches of the cervical and upper thoracic ganglia, while its parasympathetic fibers originate in the cardiac branches of the vagus and recurrent laryngeal nerves. In turn, this plexus gives rise to the **right pulmonary plexus** which in turn sends branches to the **right coronary plexus**; the **right atrial plexus** which sends branches to the **left coronary plexus**; the **left atrial plexus** and the **left pulmonary plexus** which in turn sends branches to the **left coronary plexus**.

The cardiac nerves carry both afferent and efferent fibers from both components of the autonomic nervous system. The efferent sympathetics are responsible for cardiac acceleration and dilation of the coronary arteries while the parasympathetic fibers cause slowing of the heart and coronary artery constriction.

The **pulmonary plexuses** are essentially continuations of the cardiac plexuses along the right and left pulmonary arteries. They lie on the anterior and posterior aspects of the bronchial and vascular structures at the hila of the lungs. The anterior pulmonary plexus is formed from cervical branches of the sympathetic trunk and the parasympathetic component is derived from the cardiac branches of the vagus. The posterior pulmonary plexus is formed from the outflow of the second to fifth thoracic ganglia and the parasympathetic component is derived from the cardiac branches of the vagus and the left recurrent laryngeal nerves.

From these plexuses, fibers travel with the pulmonary and bronchial vessels to supply the vascular structures, bronchi and visceral pleura. The sympathetic efferents are responsible for bronchodilatation and vasoconstriction whilst the parasympathetic efferents control bronchoconstriction, vasodilation and the secretomotor supply to the bronchial glands.

The **celiac plexus** is the largest of the autonomic plexuses and surrounds the roots of the celiac and superior mesenteric arteries at the level of T12–L1. It is located posterior to the stomach, anterior to the crura of the diaphragm and between the suprarenal glands (Fig. 3.99). Because of its relationship to the major arteries of the fore- and midgut, the distribution of the plexus is extensive and gives rise to a number of secondary plexuses – phrenic, splenic, hepatic, gastric, intermesenteric, suprarenal, renal, testicular/ovarian and superior and inferior mesenteric.

The dense network of the celiac plexus unites the two celiac ganglia which are connected to the greater splanchnic nerve carrying preganglionic sympathetic fibers from thoracic ganglia 5–10.

The **superior hypogastric plexus** sits in the extraperitoneal connective tissue, anterior to the bifurcation of the aorta, at the level of the sacral promontory. It is formed by the union of the aortic plexus with the third and fourth lumbar nerves. It divides below into right and left hypogastric nerves which descend to form the 2 inferior hypogastric plexuses. Branches from the superior plexus pass to the ureteric and testicular/ovarian plexuses and pass with branches of the common iliac arteries.

The **inferior hypogastric plexus** also lies in the extraperitoneal connective tissue but is located medial to the internal iliac arteries. It is sometimes referred to as the pelvic plexus and is formed from the hypogastric nerves and the pelvic splanchnic nerves. The plexus gives rise to secondary plexuses that are distributed with branches of the internal iliac artery – rectal, vesical, prostatic and uterovaginal.

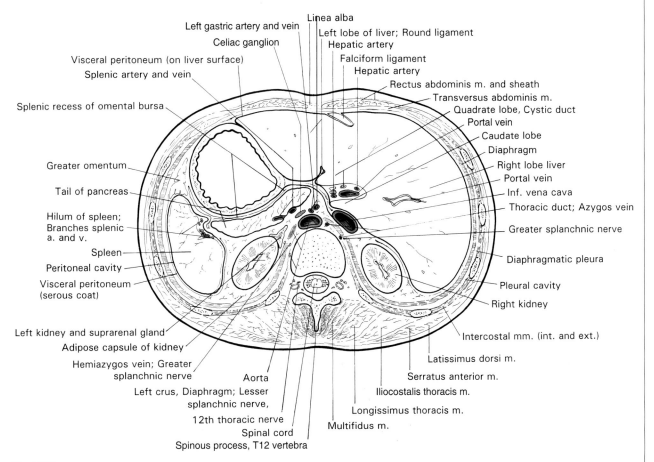

Fig. 3.99
Transverse section of the upper abdomen (level of T1) showing the relations of the celiac ganglion.

Visceral afferents

The afferent aspect of the autonomic nervous system is less well understood than the efferent distribution. Special visceral afferents occur in the olfactory nerve and in the gustatory components of the facial, glossopharyngeal and vagus nerves. Although associated with the special senses, they still elicit a visceral response, e.g. salivation at the smell of food. The remainder of visceral sensations (general visceral afferents) are separated into physiological responses which are carried in both the sympathetic and parasympathetic components and visceral pain which travels almost entirely in the sympathetic division.

Visceral afferents are derived from unipolar cells in some cranial and spinal ganglia. The cell bodies are located in the sensory ganglia of those nerves that have an autonomic efferent output (with the exception of the oculomotor nerve which carries no afferent fibers). The central processes (axons) pass in corresponding nerves into the central nervous system. For cranial nerves IX and X these fibers generally terminate in the **tractus solitarius** whilst those afferents that pass in spinal nerves pass via their dorsal roots and generally terminate in the **visceral afferent nucleus** at the base of the dorsal gray horn.

The peripheral processes (dendrites) are distributed to the appropriate viscera with the pre- and postganglionic fibers of both divisions of the autonomic system.

Physiological afferent reflex pathways

The physiological afferents generally initiate reflexes which do not reach conscious awareness. In addition, they are associated with the sensations of hunger, nausea, visceral distension, sexual sensation, etc. These general physiological sensations travel in both the sympathetic and parasympathetic divisions. General visceral afferents are conveyed from all thoracic and abdominal viscera as far distally as the splenic flexure via the **vagus** and from all more distal abdominal and pelvic viscera via the **pelvic splanchnic nerves** entering the spinal cord in the sacral region. In addition, general visceral afferents pass via **cardiac, pulmonary** and **splanchnic nerves**, with their cell bodies lying in the appropriate dorsal root ganglion. The central processes terminate in the dorsal gray matter from where impulses pass to the **intermediolateral cell column** in the lateral gray horn to initiate sympathetic efferents and so elicit a reflex action. Visceral afferents of special physiological significance travel in the parasympathetic cranial route. These include **baroreceptor** pathways from the aortic arch (vagus) and carotid sinus (glossopharyngeal) that regulate changes in arterial blood pressure. **Chemoreceptors**, are also present in the carotid body (mainly glossopharyngeal) that monitor arterial oxygen levels.

PAIN

Somatic pain

Although there is some awareness of pain at the thalamic level, it is not fully appreciated until the information reaches the cerebral cortex. Stimulation of peripheral nociceptors results in the transmission of information along a complex pathway via peripheral nerves, tracts in the spinal cord, hindbrain and midbrain to the thalamus. It is then through thalamocortical connections that the processed information reaches consciousness and perception. The final signal is interpreted as pain and it can originate anywhere along this complex path. Conscious and reflex responses to pain are modified at many points along the pathway by facilitation and inhibition at synapses.

Most sensory receptors are capable of responding to a variety of stimuli but in many cases their shape and location may dictate that they respond more efficiently to one type of stimulation than another. **Pain receptors** are typically unencapsulated free nerve endings which may have a thin myelin covering, although they are usually referred to as being unmyelinated. These nerve endings tend to branch profusely to form plexuses, so that the territories of adjacent receptors may overlap considerably. The afferent fibers from these free terminals are generally of small diameter and low conduction speed.

AFFERENT FIBERS

Fiber type	Diameter (μm)	Conduction speed (m/s)	Function
A Alpha	12–20	70–120	Proprioception, somatic motor
Beta	5–12	30–70	Touch and pressure
Gamma	3–6	15–30	Motor to muscle spindles
Delta	2–5	12–30	Pain, temperature and touch
B	<3	3–15	Preganglionic autonomic
C	0.3–1.3	0.5–2.3	Pain, reflexes, postganglionic sympathetic

In mammals, pain is transmitted through A delta and C fibers. The pain sensation conducted by the A delta fibers is the quick, sharp pain which is often described as shooting, whereas the sensation conveyed by the C fibers is slow, dull and constant.

For all areas of the body except the head and neck (see below), the peripheral processes of pain fibers (first-order neurons) pass from the receptors towards the spinal cord via the spinal nerves (Fig. 3.100). The afferent fibers pass into the **dorsal root** of the spinal nerve, and the cell bodies sit in the **dorsal root ganglia**, which are located in the intervertebral foramina where they rest on the pedicles of the vertebral arches. The central processes then pass medially and enter the **dorsolateral tract** (of Lissauer), immediately posterior to the dorsal gray horn. Here, the fibers give off collateral branches which descend in the dorsolateral tract for 1 or 2 cord segments before entering the dorsal gray horn. However, the main group of fibers ascend in the dorsolateral tract for approximately 2 cord segments before entering the dorsal gray horn. All fibers terminate in the **substantia gelatinosa** where they synapse with dendrites from the second-order neurons on the pathway. The cell bodies for the second-order neurons are located in the **nucleus proprius** (Rexed's laminae II–V) of the dorsal gray horn and their axons *cross* in the anterior white and gray commissures to form the **lateral spinothalamic tract** in the lateral funiculus of the spinal cord. As the axons cross to the opposite side, they adopt a dorsolateral position in the tract, with fibers from higher cord segments occupying a more medial position. Thus, sacral segments are represented most laterally in the tract and cervical segments more ventromedially. The spinothalamic tracts diverge in the medulla, come into close proximity in the lateral pons and eventually associate with the medial lemniscus in the rostral pons or caudal midbrain. Both tracts terminate in the ventrobasal complex of the thalamus with most fibers synapsing with the third-order neurons in the **ventral posterior lateral nucleus**.

Some pain fibers also pass in the ventral spinothalamic tract, which is the principal conduit for simple touch and pressure information. The pathway via the lateral spinothalamic tract transmits more rapidly conducting pain stimuli and produces bright, quick pain, whereas the fibers that pass in the ventral spinothalamic tract conveys dull, aching pain. Various nuclei in the thalamus are concerned with the perception and integration of pain, and although a low level of pain appreciation occurs at the thalamic level, it requires transmission of the information to the cortex before true conscious awareness is possible. Therefore, the thalamus serves as a relay and sorting station to synchronize all incoming stimuli and place them in order for correct transmission to the appropriate area

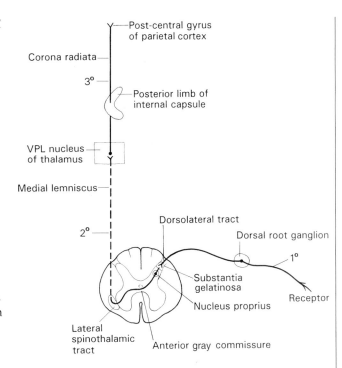

Fig. 3.100
Principal somatic pain pathway.

of the cerebral cortex. From the thalamus, impulses are conveyed via the posterior limb of the internal capsule to the post-central gyrus and posterior paracentral lobule of the cerebral cortex. However, it is not quite this simple, as pain-related information is also transferred to many other cortical areas, making the ultimate distribution of this sensation somewhat unique.

Although the spinothalamic tracts are the principal pain pathway to higher centers, pain is also conveyed to the thalamus via the spinoreticular pathway. In this way, pain may persist even after interruption of the spinothalamic tracts, as in cordotomy. The reticular formation is a diffuse, phylogenetically ancient bilateral system of polysynaptic fibers which ascend and descend throughout the spinal cord and brainstem. The reticular system of the brainstem serves to modulate the passage of impulses to the brain as all modalities pass through it and so are effectively monitored by it. The reticular formation may accentuate or inhibit impulse transmission and so act as a filter.

Trigeminal pain
The 3 divisions of the trigeminal nerve carry pain information from the region of the face, teeth, gums, sinuses, anterior scalp, etc. (Fig. 3.49). The pain fibers travel with the appropriate division of the trigeminal nerve and converge on the trigeminal ganglion on the petrous temporal ridge. The cell bodies are located here

and the central processes then pass from here into the ventrolateral region of the pons. Pain fibers descend into the spinal nucleus of the trigeminal and ultimately into the pars caudalis region (Fig. 3.50). Here, the mandibular fibers are dorsal, the maxillary fibers are central and the ophthalmic fibers are ventrally located. The second-order neurons then project to the ventral posterior lateral nucleus of the thalamus via crossed trigeminothalamic tracts. Trigeminal neuralgia (tic douloureux) presents as sporadic attacks of excruciating pain in any one or more divisions of the trigeminal nerve (but most frequently the maxillary). Trigeminal tractotomy can be performed in extreme situations and this serves to sever the connections with the lower region of the spinal nucleus in particular (pars caudalis) and so eliminate the pain fibers while leaving all the other sensory modalities relatively unaffected.

Visceral pain

Viscera are, in general, insensitive to localized pain such as cutting, burning etc. but they do confer a type of pain that is somewhat more diffuse in terms of localization and which is often described as dull or heavy. This type of pain results from distension in the viscera, tension on the mesenteries or the compression of solid viscera. Often this pain may be referred to a region of the body corresponding to the dermatome origin of the spinal nerve with which the visceral pain fibers are traveling. Hence, for example, appendicitis pain can be referred to the periumbilical region and coronary ischemia-related pain can be referred to the left side of the chest, lower neck and inner aspect of the left arm. Referred pain is that perceived by the cerebral cortex as arising in another area of the body which is not directly receiving the noxious stimulus.

Visceral pain is almost exclusively conveyed via the sympathetic component of the autonomic nervous system. These pain fibers have their cell bodies in the spinal dorsal root ganglia of T1–L3, whilst their peripheral processes reached the sympathetic trunk via white rami communicantes from the viscera via cardiac, pulmonary and splanchnic nerves. These fibers enter the dorsal gray horn of the spinal cord and terminate in the visceral afferent nucleus, which is situated laterally in the base of the dorsal horn. From here, the ascending pathways are not well defined but they may coincide with the somatic pain pathway (spinothalamic) and so reach the thalamus. Parasympathetic fibers also transmit pain from viscera in the pelvis (pelvic splanchnic nerves) and head, neck, thoracic and abdominal regions (vagus). Visceral pain tends to be projected to the insular cortex, which is associated with the autonomic nervous system and may thus produce nausea and vomiting when stimulated.

4

Anatomical regions of special interest

THORACIC INLET

The thoracic inlet is the junction between the neck and the thorax (Figs 4.1–4.3). It is bounded anteriorly by the superior border of the manubrium, posteriorly by the anterior surface of the body of the first thoracic vertebra and laterally by the medial borders of the first ribs and their costal cartilages. It is roughly kidney-shaped and slopes downwards from behind, so that the posterior wall is longer than the anterior wall.

The apices of the lungs pass upwards into the neck, covered by the dome of pleura which is in turn invested by the suprapleural membrane. Posteriorly, the lung reaches the level of the superior border of the first rib and anteriorly it extends to 3 cm above the superior border of the clavicle. The apex of the lung is grooved anteriorly by the subclavian vessels and posteriorly (from medial to lateral) by the stellate ganglion of the sympathetic trunk, the superior intercostal artery and the ventral ramus of the first thoracic spinal nerve.

The key to understanding the position of the structures at the root of the neck is to consider them in relation to the scalenus anterior muscle, as almost all of the important structures in this region are related to one of the surfaces of that muscle (Figs 4.1–4.3). The **scalenus anterior** originates from the anterior tubercles of cervical vertebrae 3–6 and passes downwards and laterally to attach to the scalene tubercle on the superior surface of the first rib. Scalenus anterior forms the lateral border of the 'triangle of the vertebral artery', with the longus colli muscle forming its medial border and the superior surface of the subclavian artery forming its base. Most of the important structures of this region are located within this triangle and are best described in relation to the scalenus anterior.

Anterior to the scalenus anterior — The **phrenic nerve** is formed at the superior aspect of the lateral border of the muscle. It descends across its anterior surface deep to the prevertebral fascia before crossing the anterior surface of the subclavian artery and the apex of the lung to enter the thorax behind the first costal cartilage. On the left-hand side, the phrenic nerve is crossed by the thoracic duct. In the upper part of the triangle, the **carotid sheath** and its contents (common carotid artery, internal jugular vein and vagus nerve) lie anterior to the scalenus anterior. However, towards the base of the triangle only the **internal jugular vein** maintains this position, as the others pass medially. The **subclavian vein** passes anterior to the muscle in a groove on the superior surface of the first rib. At the medial border of scalenus anterior it unites with the internal jugular vein to form the brachiocephalic vein. Although the subclavian artery passes behind the muscle, its **suprascapular** and

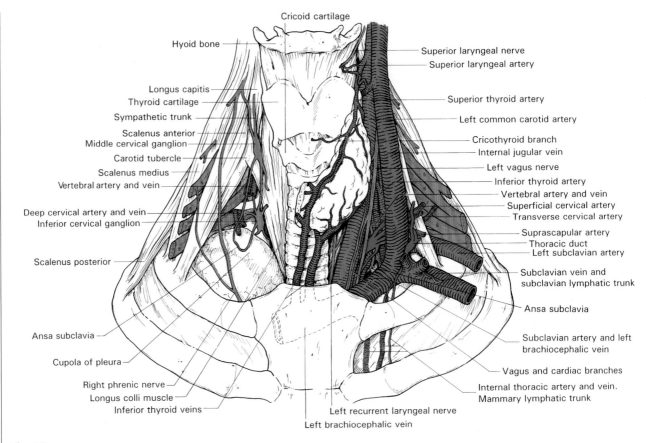

Fig. 4.1
The thoracic inlet.

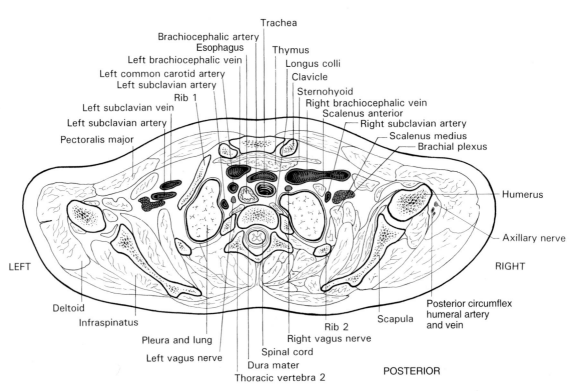

Fig. 4.2
A cross-section of the trunk at the level of the thymus.

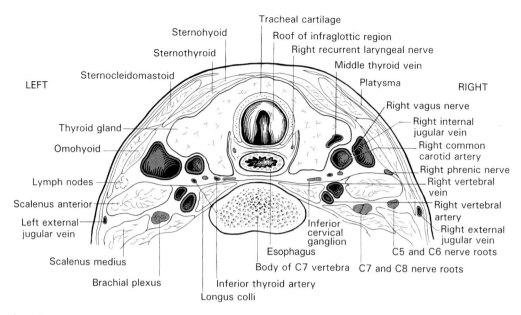

Fig. 4.3
Transverse section of the neck at the level of C7.

superficial cervical branches pass anterior to it and in so doing help to 'bind down' the phrenic nerve. The **thoracic duct** passes superiorly from the thorax to the left of the esophagus and arches laterally and posterior to the carotid sheath, anterior to the sympathetic trunk and vertebral and subclavian arteries, to enter the left brachiocephalic vein.

Posterior to the scalenus anterior—The **subclavian artery** passes behind the sternoclavicular joint, grooves the pleura and passes posterior to the middle third of the clavicle, deep to the scalenus anterior and occupies a groove on the superior surface of the first rib, anterior to the scalenus medius muscle. The scalenus anterior muscle divides the subclavian artery into 3 parts. The first part lies medial to the muscle; the second part lies behind it and the third part lies lateral to it. Only the transverse cervical branch passes posterior to the muscle, with all other branches being either anterior or medial to it. The roots of the **brachial plexus** pass posterior to the scalenus anterior behind the subclavian artery to gain access to the upper limb under the clavicle and over the superior surface of the first rib.

Medial to the scalenus anterior — The first part of

the **subclavian artery** and its branches all arise medial to the muscle. This includes the **vertebral artery** (and the vein), the **internal thoracic artery**, the **thyrocervical trunk** and the **costocervical trunk**. The **common carotid artery** and **vagus nerve** lie medial to the muscle in the lower part of the triangle. The right vagus crosses the origin of the subclavian artery posterior to the brachiocephalic vein and the sternoclavicular joint, where it gives off the recurrent laryngeal nerve which hooks around the subclavian artery and ascends in the tracheoesophageal groove. The difference in origin between the right and left recurrent laryngeal nerves can be explained by the persistence of the embryological sixth aortic arch on the left as the ductus arteriosus, whereas on the right the most inferior arch to be retained is the fourth, which forms the inferior border of the subclavian artery. The **sympathetic trunk** passes upwards lateral to the vertebral column. The stellate ganglion lies at the superior border of the neck of the first rib, posterior to the vertebral artery. The middle cervical ganglion lies anterior to the inferior thyroid artery at the transverse process of the sixth cervical vertebra and anterior to the vertebral artery.

SUMMARY OF THE STRUCTURES RELATED TO THE SCALENUS ANTERIOR MUSCLE

Anterior	Phrenic nerve	*Posterior*	Transverse cervical artery
	Thoracic duct		Roots of brachial plexus
	Carotid sheath		
	Subclavian vein		
	Suprascapular artery		
	Superficial cervical artery		
Medial	Subclavian artery		
	Common carotid artery		
	Vagus nerve		
	Sympathetic trunk		

The remainder of the structures at the root of the neck are median in position and form 4 distinct layers:

1. a superficial the **vascular** layer formed by the brachiocephalic and inferior thyroid veins (sometimes the anterior jugular)

2. an **endocrine** layer formed by the thyroid, parathyroid and thymus glands
3. a **respiratory** layer formed by the trachea and larynx
4. a deep **alimentary** layer formed by the pharynx and esophagus.

THE SCALENI MUSCLES

	Origin	Insertion
Scalenus anterior	Transverse processes of C3–C6	Scalene tubercle of first rib
Scalenus medius	Transverse processes of C1–C6	Superior border of first rib behind groove for subclavian artery
Scalenus posterior	Transverse processes of C4–C6	Outer surface of second rib

FIRST RIB

The first rib is atypical in both shape and size (Fig. 4.4). It is short, hook-like, flat and relatively broad. It has 2 articular extremities, flat superior and inferior surfaces and outer and inner borders. The head of the rib lies posteriorly and articulates via a synovial joint with the demifacet on the lateral surface of the body of the first thoracic vertebra. A slender neck passes forwards from the head and ends in the tubercle of the rib which articulates with the transverse process of the first thoracic vertebra. Between the tubercle posteriorly and the first groove on the superior surface is the site of attachment for the scalenus medius muscle.

The superior surface has a posterior groove for the passage of the subclavian artery and the lower trunk of the brachial plexus into the axilla, and an anterior groove for the passage of the subclavian vein in the opposite direction. The tubercle between the two grooves is the site of attachment of the scalenus anterior muscle. The roughened area anterior to the groove for the subclavian vein is the site of attachment for the strong costoclavicular ligament and the subclavius muscle more anteriorly. The inferior surface is unremarkable. The outer border of the rib is covered by the scalenus posterior muscle dorsally and it gives origin to the first digitation of the serratus anterior muscle behind the groove for the subclavian artery. The inner border is a site of attachment for the suprapleural membrane. The anterior extremity of the first rib articulates via its costal cartilage (primary cartilaginous joint) with the lateral surface of the manubrium.

The first rib is normally thoracic in origin but **cervical ribs** do occur and usually articulate with the last cervical vertebra. These can be either uni- or bilateral and can give rise to both vascular and neurological complications due to interference with the passage of the subclavian vessels and brachial plexus respectively.

INTERCOSTAL SPACES

These are the spaces that occur between the inferior border of one rib and the superior border of the rib immediately below (Figs 4.5–4.9). They extend from the vertebral column posteriorly and widen as they pass anteriorly to the lateral border of the sternum. The spaces are bridged by muscles and each transmits a neurovascular bundle. The importance of this area is to provide sites of attachment for the muscles that will raise the ribs on inspiration. The presence of these muscles ensures that the space is given some rigidity, so that there is no bulging of the underlying pleurae during respiration.

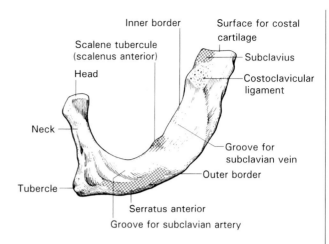

RIGHT FIRST RIB

Fig. 4.4
The right first rib.

Intercostal muscles

There are 3 types of muscle in this region:

1. those that connect adjacent ribs (intercostals, Fig. 4.5)
2. those that span several ribs (subcostals, Fig. 4.6)
3. those that attach the ribs to the sternum (transversus thoracis or sternocostals, Fig. 4.7).

There are 3 layers of **intercostal muscles** – external, internal and innermost (Fig. 4.5). There are 11 pairs of **external intercostal muscles** and these connect the inferior border of a rib with the superior border of the rib directly below. The muscle attaches close to the tubercle of the rib and the fibers pass inferomedially towards the costochondral junction where the fibers are replaced by the **external intercostal membrane**. The fibers are continuous with the external oblique muscle of the anterolateral abdominal wall. There are also 11 pairs of **internal intercostal muscles** and these lie deep to the external muscles, with the fibers running at right angles. This muscle passes from the floor of the costal groove above to the superior border of the rib below. It extends from the lateral border of the sternum as far posteriorly as the angle of the ribs where the muscle is replaced by the **internal intercostal membrane**. This muscle is continuous inferiorly with the internal oblique muscle of the anterolateral abdominal wall. The **innermost intercostal muscle** lies deep to the internal intercostal and is separated from it by the intercostal neurovascular bundle. The muscle fibers pass between the internal surfaces of adjacent ribs and tend to occupy only the middle of the intercostal space.

The **subcostal muscles** are variable both in shape and in size (Fig. 4.6). They are comprised of thin strips of muscle that pass from the internal surface of the angle

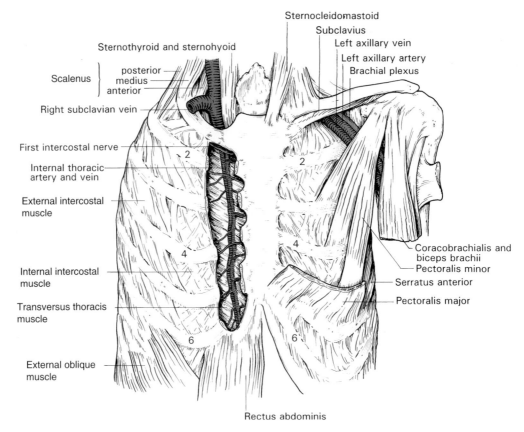

Fig. 4.5
The anterior thoracic wall.

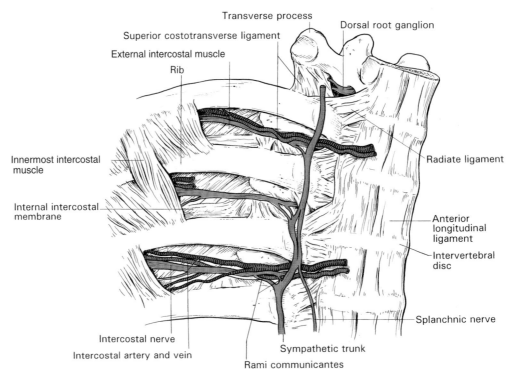

Fig. 4.6
The posterior aspect of the anterior space.

of the rib to the inferior surface of a rib that is inferior to it. Each muscle may cross 1 or 2 intercostal spaces. The fibers pass in the same inferolateral direction as the internal intercostal fibers.

The **transversus thoracis (sternocostal) muscles** consist of 4 or 5 thin strips of muscle that attach to the posterior surface of the inferior aspect of the sternum and the xiphoid process and pass superolaterally to attach to costal cartilages 2–6 (Fig. 4.7). This muscle is continuous with the transversus abdominis muscle below.

Intercostal vessels

Each intercostal space is supplied by 3 arteries and drained by at least 2 veins. The **posterior intercostal arteries** (Fig. 4.8) are derived from the descending thoracic aorta with the exception of the first, which arises from the superior intercostal artery (a branch of the costocervical trunk of the subclavian artery). As the intercostal artery approaches the posterior aspect of the space it gives off a posterior branch which accompanies the dorsal ramus of the spinal nerve to supply the skin and muscles of the back. Here, a small collateral branch is also given off which passes along the superior border of the inferior rib of that space. The main trunk of the posterior intercostal artery then passes between the parietal pleura and the internal

intercostal membrane and finally adopts a position between the internal and external intercostal muscles in the costal groove of the superior rib of that particular space (Fig. 4.9). In the costal groove, the vein lies immediately above the artery and the nerve lies directly below it. Along its course, the posterior intercostal artery supplies the muscles of that space and the underlying parietal pleura.

Two **anterior intercostal arteries** supply each space (Fig. 4.5). The arteries for the upper 6 spaces arise directly from the internal thoracic artery and those for spaces 7–9 from the musculophrenic artery (a terminal branch of the internal thoracic artery). Within each space, one anterior artery passes along the inferior border of the superior rib and the other passes along the superior border of the inferior rib. The anterior arteries of the first and second spaces pass between the pleura and the internal intercostal muscle, whilst those of the lower spaces pass between the transversus thoracis and the internal intercostal muscle. The anterior arteries eventually anastomose with the posterior arteries. However, the lowest 2 spaces do not have an anterior arterial supply but rely solely on the posterior intercostal arteries.

The **posterior intercostal veins** generally pass into the azygos and hemiazygos systems of the posterior thoracic walls and ultimately drain into the superior vena cava. The posterior veins of the first and

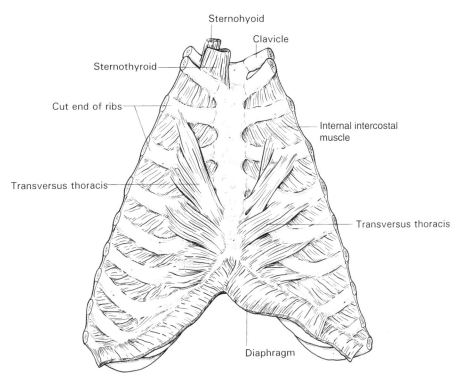

Fig. 4.7
The posterior aspect of the anterior thoracic wall.

POSTERIOR

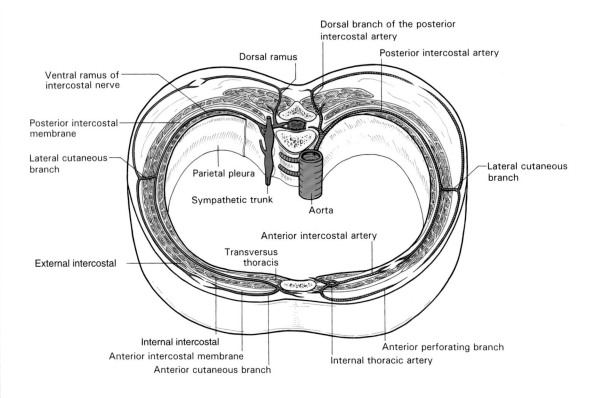

Dorsal branch of the posterior
intercostal artery

Posterior intercostal artery

Dorsal ramus

Ventral ramus of
intercostal nerve

Posterior intercostal
membrane

Lateral cutaneous
branch

Parietal pleura

Lateral cutaneous
branch

Sympathetic trunk

Aorta

Anterior intercostal artery

Transversus
thoracis

External intercostal

Internal intercostal

Anterior perforating branch

Anterior intercostal membrane

Internal thoracic artery

Anterior cutaneous branch

ANTERIOR

Fig. 4.8
Transverse section of the thorax with nerves shown on the left of the diagram and arteries on the right.

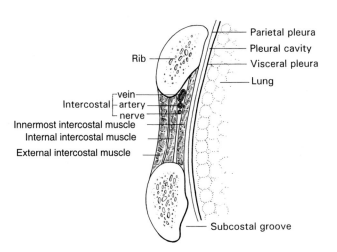

Parietal pleura

Pleural cavity

Rib

Visceral pleura

Lung

vein

Intercostal ⎱ artery

nerve

Innermost intercostal muscle

Internal intercostal muscle

External intercostal muscle

Subcostal groove

Fig. 4.9
A typical intercostal space.

sometimes second space unite to form the superior intercostal vein which may drain directly into the brachiocephalic vein. The **anterior intercostal veins** drain into the musculophrenic vein for the lower spaces, whilst the veins of the upper intercostal spaces drain directly into the internal thoracic vein which terminates in the brachiocephalic vein.

Intercostal nerves

The intercostal nerves are the ventral rami of the thoracic nerves 1–11 (Fig. 4.8). They are mixed nerves that carry both sensory and motor fibers. A typical intercostal nerve (T3–T6) enters the intercostal space between the parietal pleura and the internal intercostal membrane. At the angle of the rib it passes between the innermost intercostal and the internal intercostal to occupy the most inferior position in the costal groove. The nerve passes forwards between the internal and innermost intercostals giving branches to the muscles and underlying parietal pleura. It gives off a lateral cutaneous branch which pierces the muscles and terminates in the skin of the lateral thoracic wall. At the lateral border of the sternum the intercostal nerve turns anteriorly and pierces the overlying muscles and skin to terminate as the anterior cutaneous nerve.

The branches for a typical intercostal nerve are as follows:

1. **rami communicantes** – connection to the sympathetic trunk
2. **collateral** – intercostal muscles and pleura
3. **lateral cutaneous** – muscles and skin of lateral wall
4. **anterior cutaneous** – skin and muscles of anterior wall.

The intercostal nerve of the first space has no anterior cutaneous branch and usually no lateral cutaneous branch either. The main trunk of this nerve divides into a larger superior branch which passes into the brachial plexus and a smaller inferior branch which becomes the first intercostal nerve proper. The second intercostal nerve may also send a branch into the brachial plexus (intercostobrachial nerve) which supplies the floor of the axilla and passes with the medial cutaneous nerve of the arm to supply the medial aspect of the arm as far as the elbow joint. The intercostal nerves to the most inferior 5 spaces are thoraco-abdominal in supply, as they pass from the intercostal space into the upper part of the anterior abdominal wall.

ANTERIOR ABDOMINAL WALL

The anterior abdominal wall extends from the costal margin and xiphoid process superiorly to the iliac crest, inguinal ligament and pubic symphysis inferiorly (Figs 10A–F). Although the abdominal wall is continuous it is helpful, for descriptive purposes, to divide it into regions. This can be done in a number of ways, but there are 2 most common approaches: to divide the abdomen either into 9 regions using 2 horizontal and 2 vertical planes, or into quadrants by using 1 horizontal and 1 vertical plane (Figs 4.10A and B).

The **subcostal plane** (SCP) passes horizontally through the most inferior points of the costal margin, which generally corresponds with the 10th costal cartilage and the superior aspect of the third lumbar vertebra. The **transtubercular plane** (TTP) is a horizontal line that passes through the iliac tubercles on the crest of the ilium and corresponds with the body of the fifth lumbar vertebra. The **midclavicular lines** are vertical planes that extend from the midpoint of the clavicle to the midinguinal point.

THE REGIONS OF THE ABDOMEN (Fig. 4.10A)

Right hypochondrium	Epigastrium	Left hypochondrium
Right lumbar	Umbilical	Left lumbar
Right iliac	Hypogastrium	Left iliac

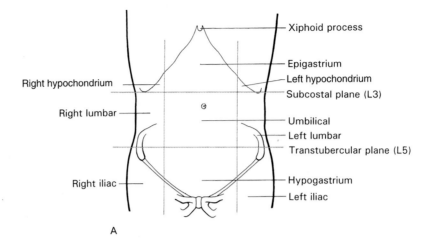

Xiphoid process
Epigastrium
Left hypochondrium
Subcostal plane (L3)
Umbilical
Left lumbar
Transtubercular plane (L5)
Hypogastrium
Left iliac
Right hypochondrium
Right lumbar
Right iliac

A

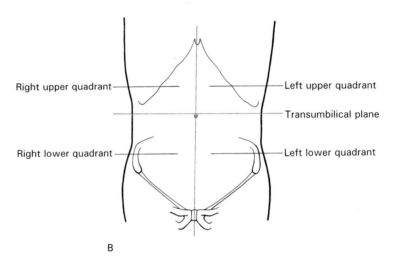

Right upper quadrant
Left upper quadrant
Transumbilical plane
Right lower quadrant
Left lower quadrant

B

Fig. 4.10 A&B
The relation of structures to the anterior abdominal wall.

Using the horizontal **transumbilical plane** which passes through the umbilicus and the **median plane** which bisects the xiphoid process superiorly and the pubic symphysis inferiorly, the abdominal wall can be separated into quadrants (Fig. 4.10B). One other useful line is the **transpyloric plane** (TPP), which is the key plane of the abdomen as so many viscera can be related to its position. The TPP is situated midway between the xiphisternal joint and the umbilicus (some texts will also state that it is midway between the jugular notch of the manubrium and the pubic symphysis) and passes through the inferior border of the first lumbar vertebra (Fig. 4.10C). The viscera that can be located along this plane are:

1. the pylorus of the stomach (hence its name)
2. the duodenojejunal junction
3. the neck of the pancreas
4. the hila of the kidneys
5. the fundus of the gall bladder
6. the origin of the superior mesenteric artery from the aorta
7. the commencement of the hepatic portal vein.

The anterior abdominal wall is essentially a muscular sheet which is formed from 4 muscles – the external oblique, internal oblique, transversus abdominis and rectus abdominis.

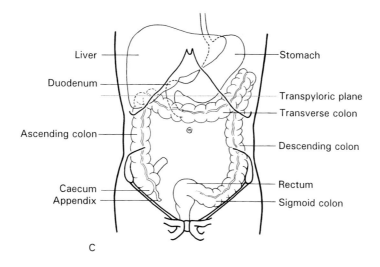

C

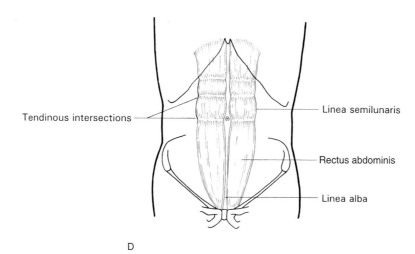

D

Fig. 4.10 C&D
The relation of structures to the anterior abdominal wall.

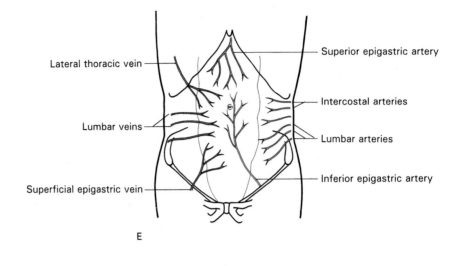

Lateral thoracic vein

Superior epigastric artery

Intercostal arteries

Lumbar veins

Lumbar arteries

Inferior epigastric artery

Superficial epigastric vein

E

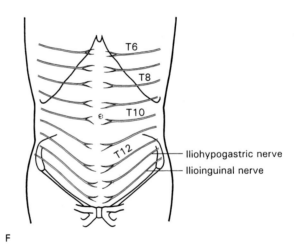

T6

T8

T10

T12

Iliohypogastric nerve

Ilioinguinal nerve

F

Fig. 4.10 E&F
The relation of structures to the anterior abdominal wall.

The **external oblique** is essentially continuous with the external intercostal muscles of the thorax and is the largest and most superficial of the muscles (Fig. 4.11A). It arises by digitations from the outer surfaces of the fifth to twelfth ribs and the fibers pass in an inferomedial direction to insert into the linea alba, the pubic tubercle and the anterior region of the iliac crest. The **linea alba** is formed by the interdigitation of the aponeuroses of the abdominal muscles of either side as they come together in the midline. On the skin surface, this area presents as a shallow depression that runs vertically from the pubis to the xiphoid process. The posterior edge of the external oblique muscle is free. At the inferior limits of the muscle, the aponeurosis is folded back on itself (rather like a roller blind) to form the **inguinal ligament**, which stretches between the anterior superior iliac spine and the pubic tubercle. The medial end of the inguinal ligament is reflected back to form the **lacunar ligament**, which attaches to the pecten pubis and its sharp free border forms the medial margin of the femoral ring. The superficial inguinal ring is a triangular defect in the aponeurosis just superior to the medial part of the inguinal ligament and transmits the spermatic cord in the male and the round ligament of the uterus in the female.

The **internal oblique** muscle lies deep to the external oblique and is continuous with the internal intercostals of the thorax (Fig. 4.11B). It arises from the thoracolumbar fascia, the anterior two-thirds of the iliac crest and the lateral half of the inguinal ligament. The fibers pass in an inferolateral direction and insert into the inferior borders of ribs 10–12, the linea alba and the pubis via the conjoint tendon. The anterior fibers also become aponeurotic and split to form the anterior and posterior walls of the rectus sheath (see below).

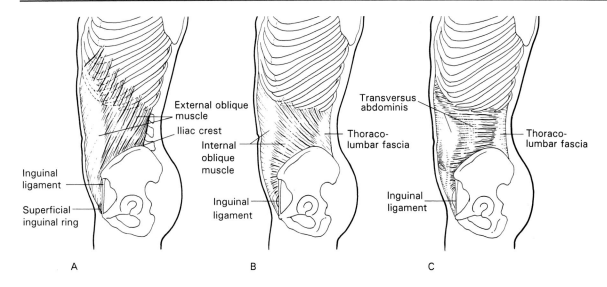

Fig. 4.11 A,B,C
The muscles of the anterior abdominal wall.

The **transversus abdominis** muscle is the deepest of the three and arises from the internal surfaces of costal cartilages 7–12, the thoracolumbar fascia, iliac crest and lateral third of the inguinal ligament (Fig. 4.11C). The fibers pass forwards in a virtually horizontal manner to attach to the linea alba, pubic crest and pecten pubis via the conjoint tendon, which is formed by the fusion of the lowest aponeurotic fibers of the transversus abdominis and internal oblique muscles.

Acting together, the 3 flat muscles can increase intra-abdominal pressure, but acting separately they serve to fix the pelvis, flex the trunk (both anteriorly and laterally, depending upon whether the muscles are working independently or as a pair) and rotate it to the opposite side.

The **rectus abdominis** arises as a narrow, thick muscle from the pubic crest and symphysis and passes upwards to attach via a broad and flat tendon to the xiphoid process and costal cartilages 5–7 (Fig. 4.12). Each rectus muscle is enclosed within its own rectus sheath and the paired recti are separated in the midline by the linea alba. The lateral border of the rectus sheath

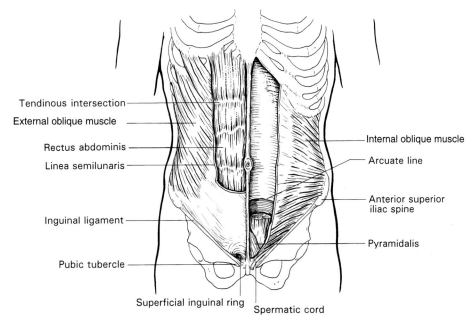

Fig. 4.12
The rectus abdominis muscle and the rectus sheath.

(linea semilunaris), passes upwards from the pubic tubercle to the tip of the ninth costal cartilage (Fig. 4.10D). The rectus sheath is formed by the aponeuroses of the 3 flat abdominal muscles (Fig. 4.13). The anterior wall of the sheath is formed from the aponeurosis of the external oblique and the anterior division of the aponeurosis of the internal oblique muscles. The anterior wall is 'bound down' to the rectus muscle by at least 3 tendinous intersections which are located:

1. just inferior to the xiphoid process
2. directly above the umbilicus
3. midway between these two points

The posterior wall of the rectus sheath is formed from the posterior division of the aponeurosis of the internal oblique and the aponeurosis of the transversus abdominis muscles. The rectus sheath is deficient superiorly at the costal margin due to the muscular attachments and it is also absent posteriorly from a point that is halfway between the umbilicus and the pubic symphysis. At this level the aponeuroses that formed the posterior wall now pass anterior to the muscle forming the **arcuate line** (Fig. 4.14). Therefore, inferior to this line, all aponeuroses of the anterior abdominal musculature pass anterior to the rectus muscle.

The contents of the rectus sheath are:

1. the rectus abdominis muscle
2. the superior and inferior epigastric vessels
3. the terminal branches of the lower 5 intercostal nerves
4. the subcostal vessels and nerves.

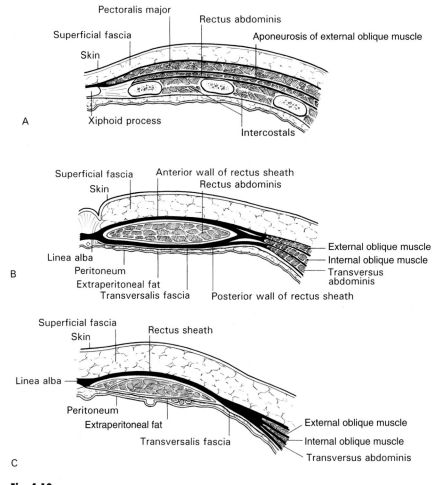

Fig. 4.13
Transverse sections through the rectus sheath. **A** Above the costal margin. **B** At the level of the umbilicus. **C** Below the level of the anterior superior iliac spine.

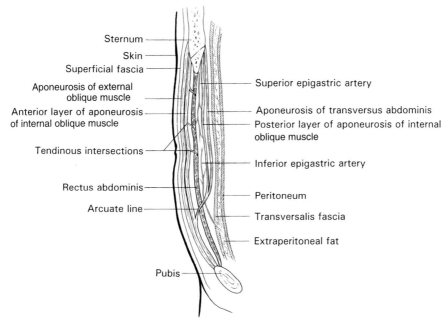

Fig. 4.14
Sagittal section through the rectus sheath.

SUMMARY OF THE ANTERIOR ABDOMINAL MUSCLES

	Origin	Insertion
External oblique	Ribs 5–12	Xiphoid process, linea alba, pubic crest, pubic tubercle, iliac crest
Internal oblique	Thoracolumbar fascia iliac crest, inguinal ligament	Ribs 10–12 and their costal cartilages, xiphoid process, linea alba, pubic symphysis
Transversus abdominis	Costal cartilages 7–12 thoraco lumbar fascia iliac crest, inguinal ligament	Xiphoid process, linea alba, pubic symphysis
Rectus abdominis	Pubic crest, pubic symphysis	Xiphoid process, costal cartilages 5–7

The main arteries of the anterior abdominal wall are the **inferior epigastric, deep circumflex iliac** and **superior epigastric arteries** (Fig. 4.10E). The inferior epigastric is a branch from the external iliac and it runs superiorly in the transversalis fascia to reach the arcuate line where it enters the rectus sheath. The deep circumflex iliac artery is also a branch of the external iliac and it runs on the deep aspect of the abdominal wall, parallel with the inguinal ligament and along the iliac crest between the internal oblique and transversus abdominis muscles. The superior epigastric artery is one of the terminal branches of the internal thoracic artery and it enters the rectus sheath below the seventh costal cartilage. The lateral aspects of the abdominal wall receive their arterial supply from the anterior and collateral branches of the posterior intercostal arteries of the lower 2 spaces, the subcostal artery and the lumbar arteries which arise from the abdominal aorta.

The venous drainage of the anterior abdominal wall passes inferiorly into the superficial epigastric vein which is a tributary of the great saphenous vein, superiorly into the lateral thoracic vein and laterally into the lumbar veins (Fig. 4.10E). In addition, the para-umbilical veins drain into the hepatic portal system.

The skin and muscles of the anterior abdominal wall are supplied by the ventral rami of the lower 5 intercostal nerves, the subcostal nerve and the iliohypogastric and ilioinguinal branches of the first lumbar nerve (Fig. 4.10F). The nerves run between the transversus abdominis and internal oblique muscles in the neurovascular plane that corresponds with their position in the intercostal spaces. The anterior cutaneous branches then pierce the rectus sheath and supply the skin as follows:

T7 – region of xiphoid process
T10 – umbilical region
T12 – midway between umbilicus and pubic symphysis
Iliohypogastric – skin over pubis
Ilioinguinal – superiomedial of thigh and external
  genitalia.

The **inguinal canal** is an oblique passage through the lower part of the anterior abdominal wall (Fig. 4.15). It allows structures to pass to and from the testis in the male and in the female it permits the passage of the round ligament of the uterus. Further, it transmits the ilioinguinal nerve in both sexes. The canal extends from the deep inguinal ring (a hole in the fascia transversalis) downwards and medially to the superficial inguinal ring (a hole in the aponeurosis of the external oblique muscle). It lies parallel to and immediately above the inguinal ligament which is the lower rolled-up border of the external oblique muscle and extends from the anterior superior iliac spine laterally to the pubic tubercle medially. The deep inguinal ring lies approximately 1.5 cm above the inguinal ligament, midway between the anterior superior iliac spine and the symphysis pubis. The superficial inguinal ring is triangular in shape, with the base formed by the pubic crest. The margins of the ring (crura) give origin to the external spermatic fascia.

The anterior wall of the canal is formed along its entire length by the aponeurosis of the external oblique muscle, which is reinforced in its lateral third by the fibers of origin of the internal oblique muscle. The posterior wall of the canal is formed along its entire length by the fascia transversalis and is reinforced in its medial third by the conjoint tendon (common tendon of insertion of the internal oblique and transversus muscles). The floor of the canal is formed by the inferior edge of the aponeurosis of the external oblique muscle (inguinal ligament) and at its medial end by the lacunar ligament. The roof of the canal is formed by the arching lowest fibers of the internal oblique and transversus abdominis muscles.

CONTENTS OF THE ABDOMINAL REGIONS

Right hypochondrium	**Epigastrium**	**Left hypochondrium**
Liver	Esophagus, liver, stomach, gall bladder (pancreas)	Spleen, stomach, left colic flexure, (liver)
Right lumbar	**Umbilical**	**Left lumbar**
Right colic flexure, ascending colon (jejunum)	Duodenum, jejunum, transverse colon, pancreas (stomach)	Descending colon (stomach, jejunum)
Right iliac	**Hypogastrium**	**Left iliac**
Appendix, caecum	Ileum, sigmoid colon, rectum	Descending colon, sigmoid colon

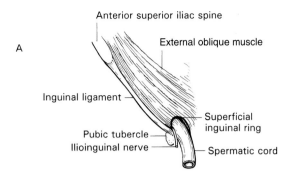

A

Anterior superior iliac spine

External oblique muscle

Inguinal ligament

Superficial inguinal ring

Pubic tubercle

Ilioinguinal nerve

Spermatic cord

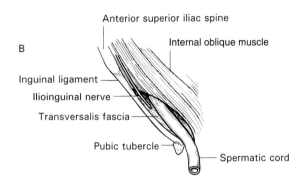

B

Anterior superior iliac spine

Internal oblique muscle

Inguinal ligament

Ilioinguinal nerve

Transversalis fascia

Pubic tubercle

Spermatic cord

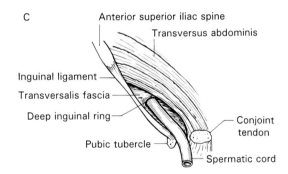

C

Anterior superior iliac spine

Transversus abdominis

Inguinal ligament

Transversalis fascia

Deep inguinal ring

Conjoint tendon

Pubic tubercle

Spermatic cord

Fig. 4.15
The inguinal canal showing the arrangement of: **A** the external oblique muscle, **B** the internal oblique muscle, and **C** the transversus abdominis muscle.

STRUCTURES PASSING THROUGH THE INGUINAL CANAL

Male

Ductus deferens
Testicular artery
Artery of ductus
deferens
Cremasteric artery
Pampiniform plexus
Sympathetic plexus
Genital branch of
genitofemoral nerve
Lymph vessels
Ilioinguinal nerve

Female

Round ligament of uterus
Ilioinguinal nerve

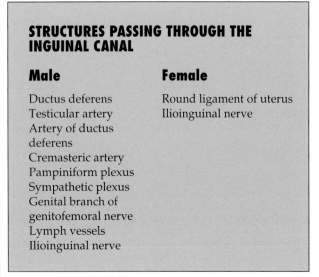

Fig. 4.16
The shape of the axilla.

AXILLA

The axilla is a pyramid-shaped space which transmits nerves, blood and lymph vessels between the root of the neck and the upper limb (Fig. 4.16). The **apex** passes upwards into the root of the neck and is bounded anteriorly by the clavicle, posteriorly by the upper border of the scapula and medially by the outer

border of the first rib. The **base** is bounded anteriorly by the anterior axillary fold (pectoralis major muscle), posteriorly by the posterior axillary fold (teres major and tendon of latissimus dorsi) and medially by the chest wall and the serratus anterior muscle (Fig. 4.17).

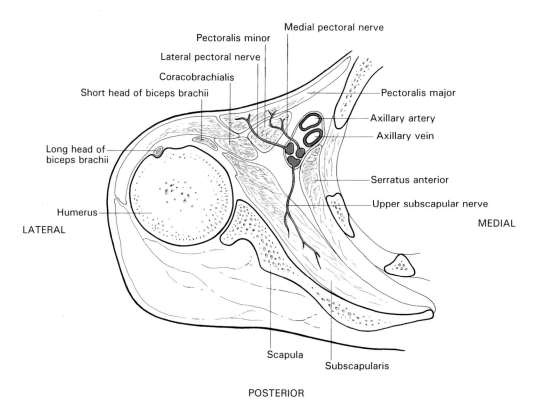

Fig. 4.17
Transverse section through the axilla.

The **anterior wall** is formed by the pectoralis major, subclavius and pectoralis minor muscles, the clavipectoral fascia and the suspensory ligament of the axilla. The **posterior wall** is formed from superior to inferior by the subscapularis, latissimus dorsi and teres major muscles. The **medial wall** is formed by the upper 5 ribs and their intercostal spaces covered by the serratus anterior muscle. The **lateral wall** is formed by the coracobrachialis and biceps brachii muscles. The **base** is formed by the skin that stretches between the anterior and posterior walls.

CONTENTS OF THE AXILLA

Axillary artery
Axillary vein
Lymph vessels and nodes
Brachial plexus

The **axillary artery** commences at the lateral border of the first rib as the continuation of the subclavian artery, and ends at the lower border of the teres major muscle, where it continues as the brachial artery. Throughout its course, the artery is closely related to the cords of the brachial plexus and their branches and is enclosed with them in a connective tissue sheath called the **axillary sheath** which is continuous superiorly with the prevertebral fascia. The pectoralis minor muscle passes in front of the artery and effectively separates it into 3 parts (Fig. 4.18):

1. The first part of the axillary artery extends from the lateral border of the first rib to the upper border of the pectoralis minor muscle and gives rise to one branch: the superior thoracic artery.
2. The second part of the artery lies behind the pectoralis minor muscle and it gives rise to 2 branches: the thoraco-acromial and lateral thoracic arteries.
3. The third part extends from the lower border of the pectoralis minor muscle to the lower border of the teres major muscle and it gives rise to 3 branches: the subscapular, and anterior and posterior circumflex humeral arteries.

The **axillary vein** is formed in the region of the lower border of the teres major muscle by the union of the venae comitantes of the brachial artery and the basilic vein. It runs upwards on the medial side of the axillary artery and ends at the lateral border of the first rib by becoming the subclavian vein.

The cords of the **brachial plexus** lie in the axilla and all 3 lie above and lateral to the first part of the axillary artery. The cords of the brachial plexus take their names from their relation to the second part of the axillary artery (Fig. 4.19). The medial cord crosses behind the artery to reach its medial side, the posterior cord lies behind it and the lateral cord lies on its lateral aspect. The important axillary branches of the brachial plexus are considered in detail in Chapter 3.

The **axillary sheath** is formed from the deep fascia that is in turn derived from the prevertebral layer of deep fascia in the neck. It encloses the axillary vessels

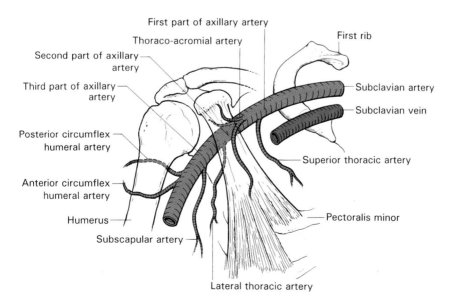

Fig. 4.18
The axillary artery and its branches.

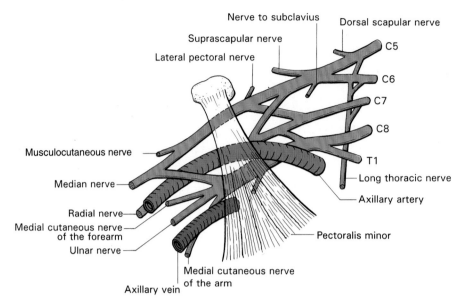

Fig. 4.19
The relations of the brachial plexus in the axilla.

and the brachial plexus. The sheath adheres to the clavipectoral fascia behind the pectoralis minor muscle and continues along the vessels and nerves as far as their entrance into the neurovascular compartment of the medial intermuscular septum of the arm.

The **axillary lymph nodes** drain the lateral part of the breast, thoraco-abdominal walls and the upper limb. They are arranged in 6 groups:

1. The anterior (pectoral) group lies along the lower border of the pectoralis minor muscle and receives lymph from the lateral part of the breast and anterolateral abdominal wall above the umbilicus
2. The posterior (subscapular) group lies in front of the subscapularis muscle and drains the back as far down as the iliac crests
3. The lateral group lies along the medial side of the axillary vein and drains most of the upper limb.
4. The central group lies in the centre of the axilla and receives lymph from the 3 previous groups
5. The infraclavicular (deltopectoral) group lies on the clavipectoral fascia in the deltopectoral triangle and drains the lateral side of the hand, forearm and arm
6. The apical group lies at the apex of the axilla and drains from all the other axillary groups. The apical nodes then drain in turn into the subclavian trunk.

On the left side, this drains into the thoracic duct and on the right into the right lymphatic trunk.

ANTECUBITAL FOSSA

The antecubital fossa is a triangular hollow situated on the anterior aspect of the elbow joint. The base of the triangle is formed from an imaginary line drawn between the medial and lateral epicondyles of the humerus. The sides of the triangle are formed from the converging borders of the pronator teres muscle medially and the brachioradialis muscle laterally. The floor of the fossa is formed from the supinator muscle laterally and the brachialis muscle medially. The immediate roof of the fossa is formed from the deep fascia, which is reinforced by the bicipital aponeurosis of the biceps brachii muscle. The roof is covered by superficial fascia and skin. Running within the superficial fascia are the basilic vein medially, the cephalic vein laterally and the median cubital vein which communicates between the other two veins (Fig. 4.20). Also found in the superficial fascia, but deep to the veins, are the branches of the medial and lateral cutaneous nerves of the forearm.

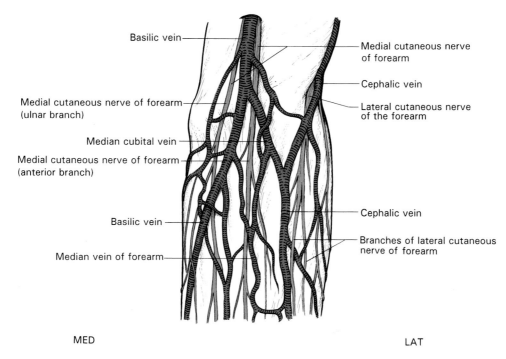

Basilic vein

Medial cutaneous nerve of forearm

Medial cutaneous nerve of forearm (ulnar branch)

Cephalic vein

Lateral cutaneous nerve of the forearm

Median cubital vein

Medial cutaneous nerve of forearm (anterior branch)

Basilic vein

Cephalic vein

Branches of lateral cutaneous nerve of forearm

Median vein of forearm

MED

LAT

Fig. 4.20
The superficial veins and nerves of the antecubital fossa.

CONTENTS OF THE ANTECUBITAL FOSSA (Figs 4.21–4.22)

(From medial → lateral)

1. The **median nerve** and its branch to pronator teres

2. The **brachial artery**, its terminal branches (radial and ulnar arteries) and recurrent branches that pass upwards to the elbow joint

3. The **tendon of the biceps brachii** passing to the radial tuberosity

4. The **radial nerve** which is found deep between the brachioradialis and brachialis muscles

5. A few **cubital lymph nodes** with efferent vessels passing from the medial aspect of the hand and forearm and afferent vessels that pass to the axillary lymph nodes

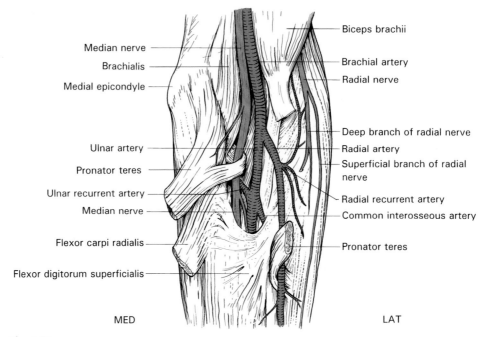

Fig. 4.21
The contents of the antecubital fossa.

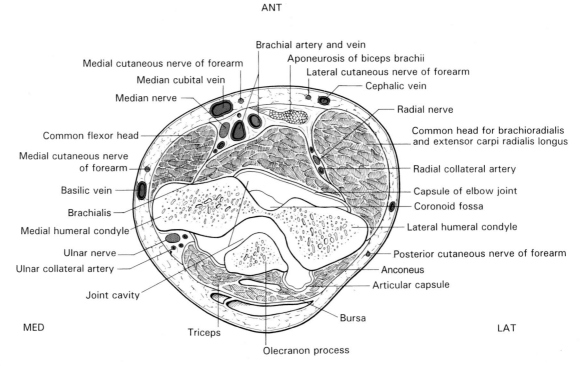

Fig. 4.22
Transverse section through the elbow joint at the level of the antecubital fossa.

Eye and orbit

The orbit is shaped like a pyramid lying on one side, with its base directed towards the face and its apex pointing back towards the middle cranial fossa. It is lined internally by periosteum (periorbita) which is a thick connective tissue that is easily detached from the roof and medial walls during surgery. This lining is continuous with the endosteal dura through various channels, including the optic canal and the superior orbital fissure. It is continuous at the orbital margin with the superior palpebral and inferior palpebral fasciae of the eyelids and with the periosteum of the bones of the face. The **orbital margin** acts as a buttress to protect the soft tissue structures housed within each orbital cavity (Fig. 4.23). The superior orbital margin is formed entirely from the frontal bone and presents a supra-orbital foramen (sometimes only a notch) in its medial third for the passage of the supra-orbital nerve and vessels. The lateral margin is formed almost entirely from the frontal process of the zygomatic bone which also shares in the formation of the infra-orbital margin. The medial orbital margin is formed superiorly by the frontal bone and inferiorly by the lacrimal crest of the frontal process of the maxilla. The orbital margin breaks its continuity at the lacrimal fossa, where the inferior margin of the orbit continues medially as the anterior lacrimal crest and the frontal bone passes medially to join the posterior crest of the lacrimal bone. These lacrimal crests delineate the bony fossa that contains the lacrimal sac on the medial wall of the orbit. The greatest diameter of the orbit lies immediately inside the rim. The volume of the adult orbit averages 30 ml whereas that of the eyeball is only approximately 6.5 ml. The depth of the orbit from the inferior rim to the optic foramen ranges from 42 to 54 mm.

Each orbit has 4 walls:
superior (roof)
medial
inferior (floor)
lateral.

The **roof** of the orbit is formed almost entirely from the thin orbital plate of the frontal bone which separates the orbit from the anterior cranial fossa and the frontal lobes of the brain. Posteriorly, the roof is formed from the lesser wing of the sphenoid bone. The frontal sinus frequently encroaches backwards into the orbital plate for a variable distance. The optic canal is located in the posterior part of the roof and transmits the optic nerve, its meninges and the ophthalmic artery. The roof is concave, especially laterally, where the lacrimal fossa accommodates the lacrimal gland.

The **medial walls** are almost parallel with each other and are separated by the superior aspect of the nasal cavities. The medial wall is paper-thin and formed by the orbital lamina of the ethmoid bone, the frontal process of the maxilla, the lacrimal bone and a small part of the body of the sphenoid bone. A vertical lacrimal groove occurs on the medial wall which is formed anteriorly by the maxilla (anterior lacrimal crest) and posteriorly by the posterior crest of the lacrimal bone. This forms a fossa for the lacrimal sac

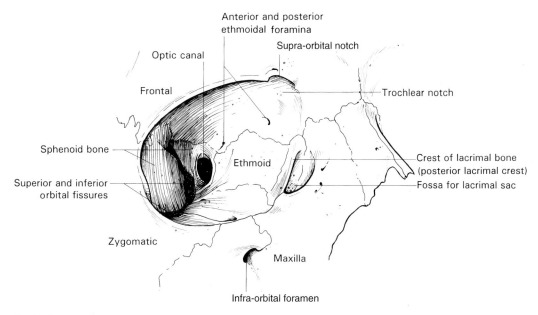

Fig. 4.23
The bony walls of the orbit.

and the nasolacrimal duct. The anterior and posterior ethmoidal foramina are also located on this wall and they transmit the anterior and posterior ethmoidal nerves and vessels.

The **floor** of the orbit slopes upwards toward the medial wall and is formed predominantly from the orbital surface of the maxilla and partly by the zygomatic bone and the orbital process of the palatine bone. The floor forms the roof of the maxillary air sinus and it is the site of the inferior orbital fissure, which transmits various structures including the infra-orbital artery and nerve. Whereas the medial wall of each orbit lies in the sagittal plane, the lateral walls lie virtually at right angles to each other.

The **lateral wall** of the orbit is thick and it separates the orbital cavity from the middle cranial fossa. It is formed from the frontal process of the zygomatic bone anteriorly and the greater wing of the sphenoid posteriorly. The roof and lateral wall are partly

separated by the superior orbital fissure, which communicates with the middle cranial fossa and transmits the oculomotor, trochlear, abducens and terminal branches of the ophthalmic division of the trigeminal cranial nerves along with the superior ophthalmic vein.

The most important contents of the orbit are the eyeball and the optic nerve, although it also contains all the extraocular apparatus, most of the lacrimal apparatus and a not insubstantial quantity of fat.

The **eyeball** occupies the anterior half of the orbital cavity while its associated muscles and nerves occupy the posterior half (Fig. 4.24). It is embedded in periorbital fat but is separated from it by the fascial sheath of the eyeball. The eye has 3 concentric coats:

1. The external or fibrous coat forms a rigid support for the eye and consists of a white, opaque posterior five-sixths called the **sclera** and a transparent anterior one-sixth called the **cornea**.

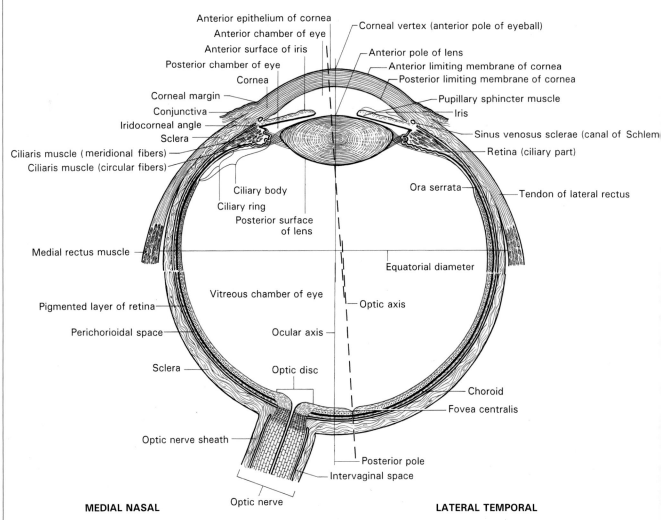

Fig. 4.24
Horizontal section of the eyeball.

2. The middle or vascular coat, which is heavily pigmented consists of, from posterior to anterior, the **choroid, ciliary body** and **iris**.

3. The inner or **retinal coat** is a thin, delicate membrane that houses the neural elements responsible for the reception and transmission of visual stimuli.

The greatest degree of visual acuity occurs at the posterior pole of the retina in the region of the **macula**. The optic nerve joins the eye medial to the macula and penetrates the entire posterior wall at the optic disc which is non-receptive and is a blind spot on the retina. The contents of the eyeball consist of the refractive media: the **aqueous humor**, the **vitreous body** and the **lens**.

A thin cup-like fascial sheath surrounds the eyeball (except for the cornea) and separates it from the periorbital fat and the other contents of the bony orbit (Fig. 4.25). The fasciae of the orbit are the **periorbita** (see above), the bulbar sheath and the muscular fasciae. The **bulbar sheath** (Tenon's capsule) is a thin membrane which covers all but the corneal region of the eyeball. It separates the eyeball from the surrounding structures and facilitates smooth movement of the eye. This sheath fuses with the sclera at the site of the optic nerve and is perforated by the ciliary vessels and nerves. Anteriorly, it is penetrated by the tendons of the ocular muscles and it is reflected as the tubular fascia onto the muscles. It fuses with the ocular conjunctiva in front of the rectus insertions leaving a small cleft known as the intervaginal space between the sheath and the sclera of the eyeball. The **fasciae of the ocular muscles** are continuous at their site of origin with the periorbita and blend anteriorly with the tubular extensions of the bulbar fascia. Fibrous extensions (medial and lateral) pass from the muscular fascia and blend with the periorbita to serve as check ligaments to restrict overactivity of the ocular muscles.

There are 7 extraocular muscles (6 move the eyeball and 1 is an elevator of the upper eyelid). The 4 recti muscles (superior, inferior, medial and lateral) derive their name from their relation to the eyeball, as they pass forwards in a cone shape to attach to the eyeball just posterior to the corneoscleral junction (Fig. 4.26). The recti all arise from a common tendinous ring (annulus tendineus) which surrounds the upper medial and lower margins of the optic canal and encircles the optic nerve. The lateral part of the ring bridges the superior orbital fissure close to its junction with the inferior orbital fissure. The superior oblique muscle lies in the upper medial portion of the orbit and runs forward to the trochlea, which is attached in the trochlear fovea of the frontal bone. The inferior oblique muscle is situated under the eyeball near the anterior margin of the orbit. These 6 muscles rotate the eyeball around 3 axes (sagittal, horizontal and vertical). The medial and lateral recti rotate the eye through the vertical axis, and so the former is an adductor and the latter is an abductor. The superior and inferior recti

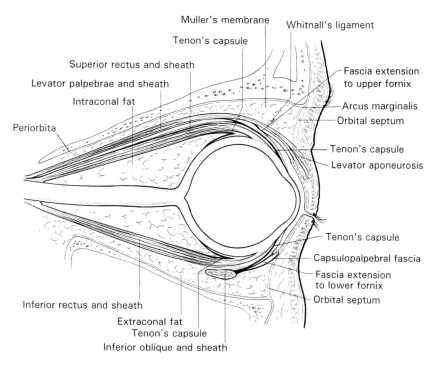

Fig. 4.25
The connective tissues of the eye.

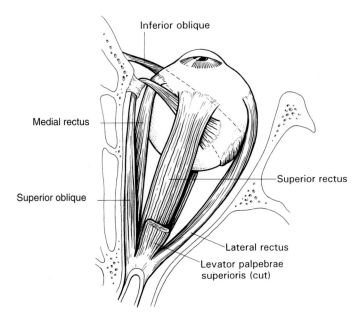

Fig. 4.26
The extraocular muscles as viewed from above.

parallel the orbital axis and not the optic axis, and so their major action is through the horizontal axis, with the former being an elevator and the latter a depressor. However, since both muscles lie medial to the centre of the vertical axis they are also adductors of the eye. As the superior and inferior recti approach the sagittal axis from the medial aspect they also produce a rotational action through the sagittal axis with the former effecting a medial (clockwise) rotation and the latter a lateral (anti-clockwise) rotation. The oblique muscles are also complex in terms of the movements they can induce. As they pass posterior to the centre of the vertical axis they both act as abductors. In the horizontal axis the inferior oblique acts as an elevator and the superior oblique as a depressor. Both muscles also cross the sagittal axis and so effect a rotational movement, with the superior oblique producing a medial and the inferior oblique a lateral rotation.

MUSCLES OF THE ORBIT

	Origin	Insertion
Levator palpebrae superioris	Tendinous ring	Skin of upper eyelid
Superior rectus	Tendinous ring	Superior and central part of eyeball
Inferior rectus	Tendinous ring	Inferior and central part of eyeball
Lateral rectus	Tendinous ring	Lateral side of eyeball
Medial rectus	Tendinous ring	Medial side of eyeball
Superior oblique	Sphenoid bone	Posterior and lateral to equator of eyeball, inferior to superior rectus
Inferior oblique	Orbital surface of maxilla	Posterior and lateral to equator of eyeball, inferior to lateral rectus

ACTIONS AND NERVE SUPPLY OF THE EXTRAOCULAR MUSCLES

	Action	**Nerve supply**
Levator palpebrae superioris	Raises upper eyelid	Oculomotor (CN III)
Superior rectus	Elevates, adducts and medial rotates	Oculomotor (CN III)
Inferior rectus	Depresses, adducts and lateral rotates	Oculomotor (CN III)
Lateral rectus	Abducts	Abducens (CN VI)
Medial rectus	Adducts	Oculomotor (CN III)
Superior oblique	Depresses, medial rotates and abducts	Trochlear (CN IV)
Inferior oblique	Elevates, lateral rotates and abducts	Oculomotor (CN III)

Orbital vessels

The principal vascular supply to the contents of the orbit is via the ophthalmic artery, although the infra-orbital artery (continuation of the maxillary artery) also offers a minor contribution via orbital branches. Venous drainage is via the ophthalmic veins (superior and inferior), which pass through the superior orbital fissure to ultimately drain into the cavernous sinus.

The **ophthalmic artery** arises from the internal carotid artery as it emerges from the cavernous sinus. It passes through the optic canal enclosed in the dural sheath of the optic nerve and runs anteriorly, close to the upper part of the medial wall of the orbit (Fig. 4.27). It then gives off several branches to structures in the orbit and to the ethmoid bone. The **central artery of the retina** is one of the smallest branches and it arises inferior to the optic nerve. It is the sole arterial supply to the retina and it runs in the dural sheath, where it pieces the optic nerve and runs with it to emerge through the optic disc. It then supplies the retina by ramifying over its internal surface. Although there is some controversy over this fact, it is generally held that these represent end arteries. Two long **posterior ciliary**

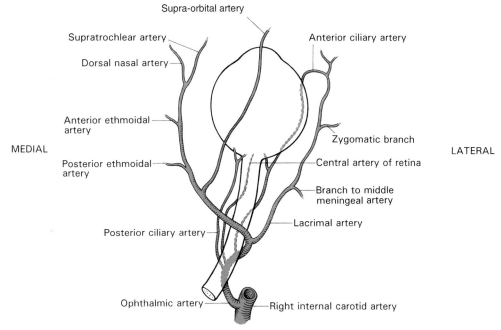

Fig. 4.27
The ophthalmic artery and its branches.

186

arteries pierce the sclera and supply the ciliary body and iris, whilst several short posterior ciliary arteries pierce the sclera and supply the choroid layer. The **lacrimal artery** is often the largest branch and it supplies the lacrimal gland, conjunctiva and eyelids via palpebral branches. **Muscular arteries** supply the extraocular muscles and these often arise from a common trunk and accompany branches of the oculomotor nerve. The muscular arteries give rise to the **anterior ciliary arteries**, which give branches to the conjunctiva and then pierce the sclera to supply the iris. The **supra-orbital**, **supratrochlear**, **dorsal nasal** and **anterior** and **posterior ethmoidal arteries** also arise from the ophthalmic artery and pass through the orbit to supply the forehead, face and nasal mucosa respectively.

The **superior ophthalmic vein** anastomoses with the facial vein and, as it is valveless, flow can be in either direction. It crosses superior to the optic nerve and passes through the superior orbital fissure to end in the cavernous sinus. The **inferior ophthalmic vein** commences as a plexus on the floor of the orbit and it communicates with the pterygoid plexus through the inferior orbital fissure. This vein crosses inferior to the optic nerve and either terminates in the superior ophthalmic vein or in the cavernous sinus. The **central vein of the retina** usually drains directly into the cavernous sinus but it may join the superior ophthalmic vein.

In contrast to the situation in most other regions of the body where arteries and veins travel together, the veins of the orbit do not accompany their arterial counterparts. Arteries radiate to their target, perforating septa as they pass through fascial compartments, whereas veins run circularly and are confined by the connective tissue septa. The greatest concentration of vessels in the posterior orbit is on the lateral aspect, whereas in the anterior orbit most vessels are placed medially, although there is enormous individual variability in the anatomical layout of the vascular system. However, the rear of the intraconal area always has a high arterial density and for this reason, along with the presence of the optic nerve, it is unwise to place a needle in the posterior 1.5 cm of the orbit.

Orbital nerves (Fig. 4.28)

Four major nerve groups enter the orbital cavity:

1. motor nerves to skeletal muscles
2. special sensory nerves to the retina (the optic nerve has been considered in Chapter 3)
3. general sensory nerves, and
4. autonomic nerves to supply smooth muscle and glandular tissue.

There are 3 motor nerves to the skeletal muscles of the orbit:

1. abducens (VI)
2. trochlear (IV), and
3. oculomotor (III).

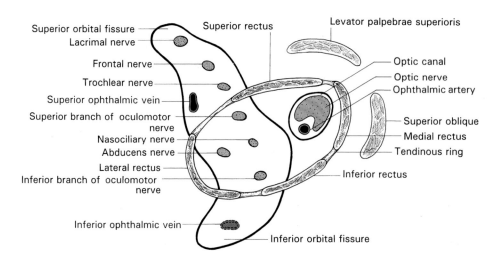

Fig. 4.28
The right superior orbital fissure and optic canal.

The **abducens nerve** enters the orbit through the superior orbital fissure and is enclosed in the tendinous ring. It innervates the lateral rectus muscle and so influences abduction of the eye. The **trochlear nerve** also enters the orbit via the superior orbital fissure but is outside the tendinous ring. It passes across the upper surface of the superior rectus and levator palpebrae superioris muscles to reach the superior border of the superior oblique muscle, which it supplies. The **oculomotor nerve** also enters the orbit through the superior orbital fissure within the confines of the tendinous ring. The nerve then separates into superior and inferior divisions, with the former supplying the superior rectus and levator palpebrae superioris muscles and the latter supplying the medial rectus, inferior rectus and inferior oblique muscles (Fig. 4.29). As the nerve enters the orbit within the tendinous ring, all the muscles are supplied from the surface that is innermost within the muscular cone. The inferior division of the oculomotor also carries preganglionic parasympathetic fibers to the ciliary ganglion (via short ciliary nerves to the sphincter pupillae and ciliary muscles).

The sensory nerves in the orbit originate from the ophthalmic division of the trigeminal nerve (Figs 4.30 and 4.31). The **frontal nerve** passes above the lateral rectus and divides into supra-orbital and supratrochlear branches to supply the skin of the upper eyelid, forehead and scalp. The **lacrimal nerve** follows the upper border of the lateral rectus nerve and ends in

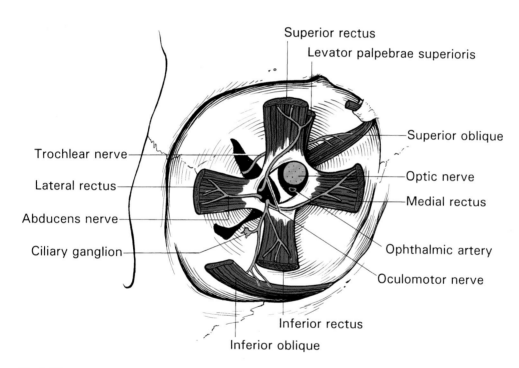

Fig. 4.29
The motor nerves of the orbit in relation to the muscular cone.

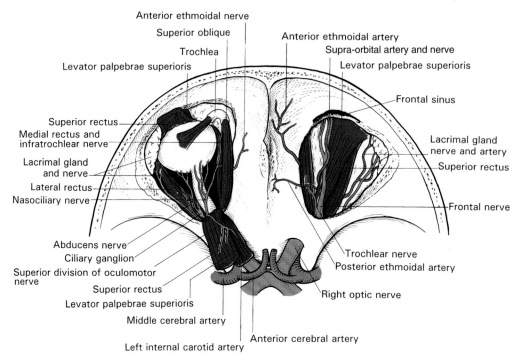

Fig. 4.30
Dissection of the orbital cavities viewed from above.

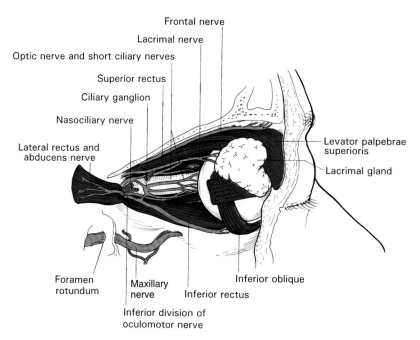

Fig. 4.31
Lateral view of the right orbital contents.

the lacrimal gland and upper eyelid. It is only sensory to the gland, as the secretomotor supply passes via maxillary nerve branches from the pterygopalatine ganglion. The **nasociliary nerve** enters the muscular cone between the two heads of the lateral rectus muscle and courses over the optic nerve to the medial wall of the orbit, where it gives rise to a number of branches including the long and short ciliary nerves. The **long**

ciliary nerves pass forwards to enter the sclera and are sensory to the eyeball. The **short ciliary nerves** are not only sensory to the eye but also carry postganglionic parasympathetic fibers from the ciliary ganglion to the smooth muscles of the eye.

Lacrimal apparatus

The lacrimal apparatus consists of the lacrimal gland, lacrimal canaliculi, the lacrimal sac and the nasolacrimal duct (Fig. 4.32). The **lacrimal gland** occupies the lacrimal fossa in the orbital plate of the frontal bone behind the superiolateral margin of the orbit. It is divided by the expanded tendon of the levator palpebrae superioris into a superior (orbital) and an inferior (palpebral) part. The lacrimal nerve conducts sensory information from the gland, whilst the secretomotor component arises in the greater petrosal nerve (preganglionic parasympathetic fibers from VII) and deep petrosal nerve (postganglionic sympathetic) and passes to the pterygopalatine ganglion. From here, postganglionic fibers travel to the gland via branches of the maxillary division of the trigeminal nerve. The **lacrimal canaliculi** occupy the margins of the eyelids from the papillae to the lacrimal sac. Each canaliculus courses towards the **lacrimal sac** which is the upper dilated portion of the nasolacrimal duct and is lodged in the vertical groove formed by the lacrimal and maxillary bones. The sac lies behind the medial palpebral ligament and in front of the lacrimal part of the orbicularis oculi muscle. The **nasolacrimal duct** extends downwards from the lacrimal sac into the inferior meatus of the nose.

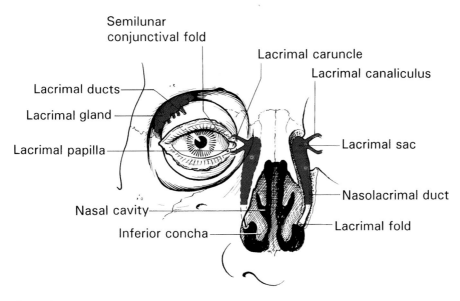

Fig. 4.32
The lacrimal apparatus.

Bibliography

Barr M L 1979 The human nervous system. An anatomical viewpoint, 3rd edn. Harper & Row, Maryland

Carola R, Harley J P, Noback C R 1992 Human anatomy. McGraw-Hill, New York

Clemente C D 1981 Anatomy. A regional atlas of the human body, 2nd edn. Urban & Schwarzenberg, Munich

Ellis H 1992 Clinical anatomy. A revision and applied anatomy for clinical students, 8th edn. Blackwell, London

Gosling J A, Harris P F, Humpherson J R, Whitmore I, William P L T 1996 Human anatomy. Colour atlas and text. Mosby-Wolfe, London

Hall-Craggs E C B 1995 Anatomy as a basis for clinical medicine. Williams and Wilkins, London

Heimer L 1995 The human brain and spinal cord, 2nd edn. Springer-Verlag, Berlin

Larsen W J 1993 Human embryology. Churchill Livingstone, New York

Moore K L 1992 Clinically oriented anatomy, 3rd edn. Williams and Wilkins, London

Rogers A W 1992 Textbook of anatomy. Churchill Livingstone, Edinburgh

Snell R S 1995 Clinical anatomy for medical students, 5th edn. Little, Brown and Company, Boston

Wilkinson J L 1992 Neuroanatomy for medical students. 2nd edn. Wright & Son, Bristol

Williams P L, Warwick R 1980 Gray's anatomy, 36th edn. Churchill Livingstone, Edinburgh

Woodburne R T, Burkel W E 1988 Essentials of human anatomy, 8th edn. Oxford University Press, Oxford

Index